OXFORD MEDICAL PUBLICATIONS

Headache

Headache : a practical manual

Published and forthcoming Oxford Care Manuals

Stroke Care: A Practical Manual
Rowan Harwood, Farhad Huwez, and Dawn Good

Multiple Sclerosis Care: A Practical Manual
John Zajicek, Jennifer Freeeman, and Bemadette Porter (eds)

Dementia Care: A Practical Manual
Jonathan Waite, Rowan Harwood, Ian Morton, and David Connelly

Diabetes Care: A Practical Manual
Rowan Hillson

Preventive Cardiology: A Practical Manual
Catriona Jennings, Alison Mead, Jennifer Jones, Annie Holden,
Susan Connolly, Kornelia Kotseva and David Wood

Oxford Care Manuals
Headache:
a practical manual

Edited on behalf of the
British Association for the
Study of Headache
by

David Kernick

General Practioner,
St Thomas Medical Group,
Exeter, UK

Peter J. Goadsby

Headache Group,
Department of Neurology,
University of California,
San Francisco, USA

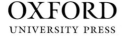

OXFORD
UNIVERSITY PRESS

OXFORD
UNIVERSITY PRESS

Great Clarendon Street, Oxford OX2 6DP

Oxford University Press is a department of the University of Oxford.
It furthers the University's objective of excellence in research, scholarship,
and education by publishing worldwide in

Oxford New York

Auckland Cape Town Dar es Salaam Hong Kong Karachi
Kuala Lumpur Madrid Melbourne Mexico City Nairobi
New Delhi Shanghai Taipei Toronto

With offices in

Argentina Austria Brazil Chile Czech Republic France Greece
Guatemala Hungary Italy Japan Poland Portugal Singapore
South Korea Switzerland Thailand Turkey Ukraine Vietnam

Oxford is a registered trade mark of Oxford University Press
in the UK and in certain other countries

Published in the United States
by Oxford University Press Inc., New York

© Oxford University Press, 2009

British Library Cataloguing in Publication Data
Data available

Library of Congress Cataloging-in-Publication-Data
Data available

Typeset by Cepha Imaging Private Ltd., Bangalore, India
Printed in Italy
on acid-free paper by
Legoprint S.p.A.

ISBN 978–0–19–923259–8

10 9 8 7 6 5 4 3 2 1

Preface

Headache can have a major impact on the lives of many people. Unfortunately, the needs of many sufferers go unmet. The objective of the British Association for the Study of Headache is to reduce this burden through education and research.

This handbook is edited by a general practitioner and an academic neurologist, both with an interest in headache, and will be relevant to all those involved in the management of headache.

We thank the members of BASH who have contributed to it, and Debbie Reinhold for her help in preparing the manuscript.

David Kernick
Peter J. Goadsby
The British Association for
the Study of Headache
www.bash.org.uk

Contents

Appendices

Detailed contents

Contributors

Ishaq Abu-Arefeh
Consultant in Paediatrics and
Paediatric Neurology
Stirling Royal Infirmary
Stirling
Consultant Paediatrician
Fraser of Allander
Neurosciences Unit
Royal Hospital for Sick Children
Glasgow

Fayyaz Ahmed
Consultant Neurologist
Hull Royal Infirmary
Anlaby Road
Hull

Anish Bahra
Consultant Neurologist
Institute of Neurology
University College London
National Hospital for Neurology
and Neurosurgery
Queen Square
London

Alex Ball
Clinical Research Fellow in
Neurology
Department of Neuroscience
University of Birmingham
Edgbaston, Birmingham

Saul Berkovitz
Consultant Physician
Royal London Homeopathic
Hospital
60 Great Ormond Street
London

Mike Cummings
Medical Director and Honorary
Clinical Specialist
British Medical Acupuncture
Society
Royal London Homeopathic
Hospital
London

Brendan Davies
Consultant Neurologist & Clinical
Director
North Midlands Regional
Headache Clinic
Department of Neurology
University Hospital of North
Staffordshire
Stoke-on-Trent

Paul Davies
Consultant Neurologist
Department of Neurology
Northampton General Hospital
Northampton

Andrew Dowson
Director of the King's Headache
Service
King's College Hospital
Denmark Hill
London

Giles Elrington
Consultant Neurologist
Bart's and the London NHS Trust
London

Manuela Fontebasso
General Practitioner with a special
interest in Headache
Headache Clinic
Department of Neurosciences
York Hospital
York

John Fox

General Practitioner with a special interest in Headache
St Thomas Health Centre
Cowick Street
Exeter

Nicola Giffin

Consultant Neurologist
Department of Neurology
Royal United Hospital
Bath

Peter J. Goadsby

Headache Group
Department of Neurology
University of California
San Francisco
USA

Ibrahim Imam

Neurology Specialist Registrar
Derriford Hospital
Plymouth

Ronald S Kaiser

Clinical Associate Professor
Department of Neurology
Consulting Psychologist
Jefferson Headache Center
Thomas Jefferson University
Philadelphia
Pennsylvania
USA

David Kernick

General Practitioner
St Thomas Health Centre
Exeter

Hisham Khali

Consultant ENT Surgeon
Derriford Hospital
Plymouth
Honorary Clinical Senior Lecturer
Peninsula College of Medicine and Dentistry
Plymouth

Anne MacGregor

Director of Clinical Research
The City of London Migraine Clinic
London

Manjit Matharu

Senior Lecturer and Honorary Consultant Neurologist
Institute of Neurology
University College London
National Hospital for Neurology and Neurosurgery
Queen Square
London

Suzanne O'Leary

Specialist Registrar Radiology
South West Training Scheme
The Royal Cornwall Hospital
Truro

Christopher Price

Specialist Registrar in Neurology
Royal Devon and Exeter Hospital
NHS Foundation Trust
Exeter

Bhola Ria

Headache Nurse
Institute of Neurology
University College London
National Hospital for Neurology and Neurosurgery
Queen Square
London

Alison Sentance

Headache Physiotherapy Practitioner
Physiotherapist
St George's Healthcare NHS Trust
London

Nick Silver

Consultant Neurologist
The Walton Centre for Neurology and Neurosurgery
Lower Lane
Liverpool

Tom Sulkin
Consultant Radiologist
The Royal Cornwall Hospital
Truro

Stuart Weatherby
Consultant Neurologist
Department of Neurology
Derriford Hospital
Plymouth

Tom Whitmarsh
Consultant Physician
Glasgow Homeopathic Hospital
Regional Services
North Glasgow Division
Greater Glasgow Health Board
Glasgow

Abbreviations

±	plus or minus
≤	less than or equal to
≥	more than or equal to
~	approximately
°	degrees
ACE	angiotensin-converting enzyme
ANF	antinuclear factor
APPT	activated partial prothrombin time
AVM	arteriovenous malformation
bd	twice a day
BoNTA	botulinum toxin type A
BP	blood pressure
BPPV	benign paroxysmal positional vertigo
CADASIL	cerebral autosomal dominant arteriopathy with subcortical infarcts and leukoencephalopathy
CBT	cognitive-behavioural therapy
CCH	chronic cluster headache
CECT	contrast-enhanced CT
CGH	cervicogenic headache
CH	cluster headache
CHC	combined hormone contraception
CNS	central nervous system
COC	combined oral contraceptive
CPAP	continuous positive airway pressure
CPH	chronic paroxysmal hemicrania
CRP	C-reactive protein
CSF	cerebrospinal fluid
CT	computed tomography
CVA	cerebrovascular accident
CVT	central venous thrombosis
DMPA	depot medoxyprogesterone actetate
DVT	deep vein thrombosis
EBM	evidence-based medicine
ECG	electrocardiograph
ECH	episodic cluster headache
EDH	extradural haematoma
EEG	electroencephalograph

EMG	electromyograph
EPH	episodic paroxysmal hemicrania
ESR	erythrocyte sedimentation rate
FBC	full blood count
FHM	familial hemiplegic migraine
GBM	glioblastoma multiforme
GCS	Glasgow Coma Score (Scale)
GnRH	gonadotrophin-releasing hormone
GON	greater occipital nerve
GP	general practitioner
HC	hemicrania continua
HIV	human immunodeficiency virus
HRT	hormone replacement therapy
HSV	herpes simplex virus
5-HT	5-hydroxytryptamine
IHS	International Headache Society
IIH	idiopathic intracranial hypertension
IM	intramuscular
INR	international normalized ratio
IUD	intrauterine device
IUS	intrauterine system
IV	intravenous
LFT	liver function test
LP	lumbar puncture
MA	migraine with aura
MELAS	mitochondrial encephalamyopathy, lactic acidosis and stroke-like episodes
MO	migraine without aura
MRA	magnetic resonance angiography
MRI	magnetic resonance imaging
MRV	magnetic resonace venography
NLP	neuro-linguistic programming
NSAID	non-steroidal anti-inflammatory drug
NTIS	National Teratology Information Service
od	once daily
ONS	occipital nerve stimulation
PCR	polymerase chain reaction
PET	positron emission tomography
PFO	patent foramen ovale
PGD	patient group direction
PH	paroxysmal hemicrania

PO	per os
POM	prescription-only medicine
POP	progesterone-only pill
PR	per rectum
PTH	post-traumatic headache
PTSD	post-traumatic stress disorder
PV	plasma viscosity
QALY	quality-adjusted life year
RCT	randomized controlled trial
RSVS	reversible segmental vasoconstriction syndrome
SAH	subarachnoid haemorrhage
SC	subcutaneous
SDH	subdural haematoma
SHM	sporadic hemiplegic migraine
SIH	spontaneous intracranial hypotension
SLE	systemic lupus erythematosus
SSRI	selective serotonin re-uptake inhibitor
SUNCT	short-lasting unilateral neuralgiform headache attacks with conjunctival injection and tearing
TAC	trigeminal autonomic cephalalgia
TB	tuberculosis
TCA	tricyclic antidepressant
TCH	thunderclap headache
tds	three times a day
TIA	transient ischaemic attack
TMD	temporomandibular disorder
TTH	tension-type headache
VAS	visual analogue scale

Getting to grips with the basics

Headache impact

Headache prevalence and incidence

Epidemiological estimates depend on the population studied, sampling methodology and diagnostic criteria used. Studies seek to measure:

- Prevalence—the proportion of a given population that has a disorder over a defined period of time, usually one year. The most prevalent headaches across different settings are:
  - Community—tension type (70% of the population in one year)
  - Primary care—migraine (70–90% of headache consultations)
  - Secondary care—migraine (>75% of headache consultations)

Table 1.1 shows some estimates of headache lifetime prevalence in the population.

- Incidence—the onset of new cases of a disease in a defined population over a given period of time, usually one year. Table 1.2 show the annual incidence of some important secondary headaches.

Headache impact

- 4% of the population report headache on more that >15 days each month, with rates in women higher.
- Global impact. Headache is common in all countries. Migraine is in the World Health Organization (WHO) top 20 in terms of disability-adjusted life years (a measure of the degree of disability and time spent with it). If other types of headache are included, headache is likely to be in the top 10 and in the top 5 for females (see Table 1.3).
- Impact in the workplace
  - In the UK each year, migraine sufferers lose 5.7 working days.
  - 25 million days are lost from work or school in addition to reduced performance.
  - The overall loss of productivity due to migraine has been estimated at >£2 billion a year in the UK and US$19.6 million in the USA.
- Impact on the family
  - 50% of migraineurs feel they are more likely to argue with their partners and children because of their problem.
  - A third believe they would be better partners but for their headaches.
- Impact on the individual. The well-being of migraine patients is impaired between as well as during attacks.
  - In the UK, 5.85 million people aged 16–65 are affected and experience 190 000 attacks everyday.
  - 85% report reductions in their ability to do household work and chores.
  - 45% miss family, social and leisure activities.
  - 32% avoid making plans for fear of cancellations.

Table 1.1 Estimated lifetime prevalence of headache

Headache type	Prevalence (%)
Primary headache	
Tension-type headache	78%
Migraine	16%
Cluster	0.3%
Secondary headache	
Fasting	19%
Nose/sinus disease	15%
Head trauma	4%
Non-vascular intracranial disease	0.5%
Vascular intracranial disease	0.5%

Table 1.2 Estimates of annual incidence of some important secondary headaches

Cause of headache	Incidence per 100 000 population per year
Subarachnoid haemorrhage	10
Bacterial meningitis	3
Viral meningitis	11
Temporal arteritis	10
Primary brain tumour	8

Table 1.3 World Health Organization leading causes of years with disability (both sexes age 15–44)

Disability	Rank	Disability	Rank
Depressive disorders	1	Congenital abnormalities	11
Deafness	2	Perinatal conditions	12
Anaemia	3	Alzheimer's	13
Chronic obstructive pulmonary disease	4	Dementias	14
Alcohol disorders	5	Road traffic accidents	15
Osteoarthritis	6	Malnutrition	16
Schizophrenia	7	Cerebral vascular disease	17
Falls	8	HIV/AIDS	18
Bipolar affective disorders	9	**Migraine**	19
Asthma	10	Diabetes	20

- Quality of life in migraine is similar to that of patients with other chronic conditions such as arthritis and diabetes, and worse than that of those with asthma.

Addressing the unmet need

Despite considerable impact, the needs of headache sufferers are often unmet.

- 3% of the adult population will consult for headache with their GP each year.
- Diagnosis is incorrect in at least a third of cases.
- 4% of GP headache consultations will result in referral to secondary care.
- Headache referrals represent >30% of neurological referrals.
- 50% of migraineurs are satisfied with their current treatment.
- Fewer than 10% of migraineurs are under regular medical review.
- The majority of migraineurs self-medicate.
- A review of 500 hospital attendances by a headache patient organization found that:
  - 21% of patients were not given the opportunity to ask questions or discuss their concerns.
  - 39% felt that their condition was not fully explained to them.
  - 35% felt disappointed.
  - 11% left the consultation angry!

The reasons for these failures of care are not known, but may include:

- The fact that the mechanisms of headache are poorly understood
- The subjective and intermittent nature of the problem
- A degree of stigmatization due to an association with anxiety and depression
- Poor training in headache medicine

In conclusion, there are a number of barriers to addressing the unmet needs of headache that include failure of sufferers to seek medical attention, lack of acknowledgement of the problem, and practitioners who lack the time or skills to deal with the problem adequately

Table 1.4 An example of the impact of headache in the workplace

A study in an NHS Trust hospital in Hull suggested:

- 20% of respondents experienced disabling headache each year
- The average was 16 migraine attacks per year
- The average work loss was 2 days a year, with considerably reduced efficiency at other times.
- The annual financial cost to the Trust was £100 000
- 78% of respondents were using non-prescription medication.

Mountstephen A, Harrison R (1995). A study of migraine and its effect in a working population. *Occupational Medicine.* **45:** 311-7.

Table 1.5 An example of the personal cost of headache

'I lead a busy professional, family and social life and when I get migraine the only relief for me is to go to bed and hope for sleep. This is not often possible and as such my life and work is disrupted and I often have to let my family down. At work I try and work through my migraine but I am conscious that I am not working to the best of my ability. I sometimes vomit uncontrollably, which can be embarrassing. No medication seems to help and I find doctors generally uninterested, so there seems little point in returning to my GP or complaining, as I am told nothing can be done about them. I therefore have accepted migraine as part of my life for now and hope that with age, things will improve'. (A migraine sufferer)

The classification of headache

For 95% of headaches the underlying mechanisms are not fully under-stood. Here the emphasis is on description and classification. This is an important first step to help understand underlying pathophysiology, and to predict outcome and response to therapy.

The modern era of classification began at the turn of the 19th century when symptoms and signs were linked with the appearance of organs after death. This approach was later supplemented by bacteriological and biochemical criteria. By necessity, the classification of many headaches is based on observation and, in part, response to specific treatment. As such, many diagnostic categories are decided by committee.

The International Headache Society Classification

- The first formal classification was undertaken by the International Headache Society in 1988 and updated in 2004.
- In primary care, 95% of headaches will be primary (no demonstrable cause) and 5% secondary (a demonstrable cause). There is a complex interplay of genetic and contextual factors that operate in headache, making descriptive classification in primary headaches problematic (see Fig. 1.1).

Main primary headaches
- Migraine
- Tension-type headache
- Cluster headache and other trigeminal autonomic cephalalgias

Main secondary headaches
- Headache attributed to head or neck trauma
- Headache attributed to cranial or cervical vascular disorder
- Headache attributed to non-vascular intracranial disorder
- Headache attributed to a substance or its withdrawal
- Headache attributed to infection
- Headache attributed to disorder homeostasis
- Headache or facial pain attributed to disorder of cranium, neck, eyes, nose, sinus, teeth, mouth or other facial or cranial structures
- Headache attributed to psychiatric disorder
- Cranial neuralgias and central causes of facial pain.

See Appendix 1 for a more detailed list and (www.i-h-s.org) for a full list.

Table 1.6 An example of formal IHS diagnostic criteria. In clinical practice, criteria are relaxed.

The diagnostic criteria for migraine without aura are:

A. At least 5 attacks fulfilling criteria B–D

B. Headache attacks lasting 4–72h (untreated or unsuccessfully treated)

C. Headache has at least two of the following characteristics:
  - Unilateral location
  - Pulsating quality
  - Moderate or severe pain intensity
  - Aggravating or causing avoidance of routine physical activity

D. During headache, at least one of the following:
  - Nausea and or vomiting
  - Photophobia and phonophobia

E. Not attributed to other disorders (a formal diagnosis of migraine therefore must include an examination to exclude another disorder.)

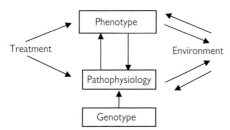

Fig. 1.1 Genetic and environmental factors that interplay to produce the headache and its characteristics. The headache in turn feeds back and influences physiological and environmental change.

Chronic daily headache

This is a descriptive definition, i.e. headache that occurs on 15 or more days of the month.

- Although clinically the term is still in widespread use, it is not recognized by the IHS classification and should be used only as an initial diagnosis in an attempt to start to evaluate a patient.
- The underlying diagnosis should be clarified. For example, medication overuse headache, chronic migraine, chronic tension-type headache, hemicrania continuum.

Formal and practical criteria

- Although the IHS criteria are rigorously applied for headache research, from a clinical perspective, a more pragmatic approach is invariably adopted. In migraine, a number of pragmatic criteria have been devised that have high levels of sensitivity and specificity (see Table 1.7).
- The current classification that attempts to force patients into a diagnostic box on the basis of clinical presentation could inhibit our understanding of primary headache.

Table 1.7 Examples of pragmatic criteria for migraine diagnosis with high sensitivity

Features	Likelihood ratio (confidence intervals)
• Headache causes disability • Nausea • Sensitivity to light	3.2 (2.7–3.9) Lipton (2003)
• Pulsating • Duration 4–72h • Unilateral • Nausea • Disability	24 (1.5–388) Detsky (2006)

Lipton R (2003). A self administered screen for migraine in primary care: the migraine ID validation study. *Neurology.* **61:** 375-382.

Detsky M, *et al.* (2006). Does this patient with headache have a migraine or need neuro imaging? *JAMA.* **296:** 1274-1283.

Developing evidence-based headache care

The evidence-based medicine (EBM) movement seeks to integrate the best scientific research evidence with clinical expertise to address four questions:

- Efficacy—what works in the research setting?
- Effectiveness—what works in the setting in which the intervention is to be delivered?
- Efficiency—what effective treatments are worth paying for against a background of limited health care resources?
- Equity—is the intervention accessible to all groups of patients?

The four steps of EBM are shown in table 1.8.

Current policy views evidence as a hierarchy of validity that sees meta-analysis of randomized controlled trials (RCTs) as the gold standard (see Table 1.9)

Challenges in headache research

Obtaining a rigorous evidence base in headache remains problematic, and in many cases diagnosis and treatment are based on clinical experience. This is because:

- Pathophysiology is poorly understood.
- There are no specific diagnostic tests.
- Treatment outcomes are subjective.
- High placebo rates in studies: 30–40% in adults and up to 60% in children.
- Clinical trial settings do not relate to real life settings. For example, acute intervention studies require patients to wait until their pain is moderate to severe before medication is taken, and that no other drugs can be taken during the attack.
- Clinical trials are expensive to undertake and mainly focused on drugs with good investment prospects. Many existing drugs are unlikely to be formally tested.
- Publication bias. As in other clinical areas, the majority of studies are promoted by the pharmaceutical industry where there is a natural tendency to publish favourable studies at the expense of those that may not show products in such a positive light.

Headache outcome measures

- Outcome measures can be used to prioritize competing resource claims, screen for unmet need, facilitate communication between patient and physician, support clinical audit and monitor response to treatment.
- Headache outcomes are difficult to measure due to the subjective nature of the condition.

Table 1.8 The four steps of evidence-based medicine

- Turn information needs into focused, answerable, clinical questions
- Locate the evidence
- Appraise the evidence for validity and usefulness
- Interpret the evidence and apply it to the patient

Table 1.9 Current hierarchy of evidence

- Meta-analysis of high quality trials
- Multicentred RCT
- Single-centre RCT
- Historic control
- Case–control
- Database analysis
- Case series
- Expert opinion

Acute therapy
- In practice, patients will trade-off a number of benefits that include speed of onset, effectiveness of pain relief, incidence of recurrence, side effects and ease of administration.
- The current primary outcome measure is the proportion of attacks effectively stopped (headache from moderate to severe to mild or no headache within a set time).
- Secondary outcome is time to meaningful relief.

Preventative therapy
- The main outcome is number of attacks over a defined period such as 3 weeks.

Placebo
- Placebos may be activating similar pain-modulating brain structures as active drugs.
- Due to the magnitude and wide range of placebo responses it can be difficult to compare studies.
- One option is to calculate the therapeutic gain, i.e. the actual response rate less the placebo response rate. However, this assumes that the effects of placebo and active elements are additive.

Measuring quality of life
- The recognition that the burden of illness cannot be fully described by clinical measures alone has led to the development of health-related quality of life measurements.
- An emerging consensus suggests that both generic (designed to be applicable to all population subgroups and useful for comparing outcomes between them) and disease-specific (designed to be applicable to one group and useful in detecting changes in the condition) measures should be administered.
- The three main theoretical approaches to measuring quality of life are shown in Table 1.10.

Qualitative research

More recently, there has been an increasing acceptance of qualitative approaches that encompass a number of methodologies.
- This involves the collection, analysis and interpretation of data that are not readily reduced to numbers.
- Data relate to the social world and the concepts and behaviours of those within it as they make sense of the situation they find themselves in.
- The focus is on exploring and understanding meaning, and the interpretation of phenomena.
- Although in theory qualitative methods would be a valuable resource in headache research, to date very few papers have been published in the area.

Table 1.10 Approaches to the measurement of quality of life

1. Quality of life is considered as the gap between experience and expectation—patients with severe disability will not necessarily report a poor quality of life.
2. Values are assigned to health states based on judgements. These are underpinned by the concepts of risk and sacrifice, and derive utility values between 0 (equivalent of death) and 1 (perfect health). For example, the quality-adjusted life year (QALY).
3. Models are used that consider domains of human existence. For example, social, psychological and physical domains. E.g. Short Form36

Table 1.11 Consumers' involvement in headache research

- Some advantages claimed for involving consumers in research:
  - Can ensure that issues that are important to consumers and therefore to the health service are identified and priortized
  - Helps to ensure that research doesn't just measure outcomes that are identified and considered important by professionals.
  - Can help with recruitment.
  - Can disseminate results of research and work to ensure that changes are implemented.
  - Ensure that the views of all relevant stakeholders are equally considered.
- There is increasing recognition that the relevance of much research falls short of patients' needs, and priorities do not always reflect the views of all relevant stakeholders.
- Traditionally, patients have been involved in research as subjects but not as equals.
- Patients as both service users and citizens have the experience and skills that can complement those of the researcher and have relevant ideas about which research questions are worth asking and judging the findings.

The headache consultation

- In the UK, 3% of GP consultations are for headache, of which 4% are referred to secondary care.
- 30% of neurology consultations are for headache.
- In all settings, migraine is the most common diagnosis. One large multicountry study found that migraine accounted for >90% of recurrent headache presenting to primary care.
- For primary headaches, cure is rarely possible. The aim is to change the locus of control from a situation where the headache invariably has control over the sufferer to one where the patient has an understanding of and control over their problem.
- Effective physician–patient communication improves patient health outcomes. As the headache presentation contains physiological, motivational, affective and cognitive components, optimum management is likely to include a number of dimensions that include pharmaceutical, social, psychological and behavioural factors.

Table 1.12 shows what patients want from a consultation. These needs may be difficult to address within the constraints of a GP consultation. Table 1.13 offers some factors that can facilitate the process and improve outcomes.

The history

The history is the most important diagnostic tool, as invariably examination will be normal. Important questions are:

- How many types of headache do you have? Often patients will recognizse more than one type of headache, and this can cause diagnostic confusion if these are not considered individually. Clinically it is most rewarding to focus on the type that gives most distress at least in the first encounter.
- Circumstances and age of onset:
  - Migraine invariably starts in childhood or early adult life.
  - Migraine and cluster can be triggered by head trauma.
  - Peripartum period—cortical vein or sagittal sinus thrombosis.
  - New presentation over the age of 50 more frequently has a secondary cause—temporal arteritis is the most common.
- Location—radiation
  - Migraine is usually unilateral. Cluster is almost always unilateral.
  - Tension headache is usually bilateral.
  - Focal pain alerts to the possibility of local pathology.
- Severity and quality
  - Patients can describe pain on a scale from 0 (no pain) to 10 (the worse pain imaginable). This can be useful for diagnosis and monitoring of treatment.

Table 1.12 What do headache patients want from their consultation?

- To be taken seriously by a sympathetic doctor—witnessing suffering is an important therapeutic tool.
- To have their ideas, concerns and expectations explored.
- To have their problem explained in terms they understand.
- To be offered informed choice about treatment
- They do not want to be abandoned. Follow-up is important; <10% of migraineurs are under continuing care.

Table 1.13 Some things that may facilitate the consultation

- Allow patients to describe their headaches spontaneously without interruption—this alone allows a correct diagnosis in 60% of headaches. (The average time a patient is allowed to talk before interruption is 18s. Without interruption, it is 150s.)
- Patients have difficulty communicating the impact of their problem. Use headache impact scores (see Appendix 2).
- Ask the patient to keep a headache diary. This is helpful for diagnosis and allows the practitioner a little extra time. Include prescribed and non-prescribed medication.
- If the consultation is anticipated, ask the patient to write down what they think is the cause of their problem and what they are hoping to get out of the consultation.
- Write a clear management plan. If in specialist care, copy the GP letter to the patient. Preferably write to the patient and copy the GP.
- Supply or direct to written educational material.
- Direct to patient support groups
- Recognize those at risk for ineffective communication: the elderly, lower socio-economic background, poor health status.

Table 1.14 Think where the headache is coming from

- Stretching of the dura due to raised CSF pressure, e.g. cough headache, idiopathic intracranial hypertension,
- Stretching of the dura or cranial nerves due to a space-occupying lesion,
- Invasion of the dura, e.g. tumour,
- Meningeal inflammation, e.g. meningitis, blood in the CSF.
- Pain arising from structures outside the skull, e.g. muscle, artery and sinus

- The pain of cluster headache is excruciating—often described as if a red hot poker is being driven into the eye.
- Migraine is very often described as throbbing or pulsatile.
- Brain tumour and meningitis are usually constant.
- Tension type is dull, nagging and persistent 'like a band'.
- An acute 'thunder clap headache' (TCH) can be caused by subarachnoid haemorrhage (SAH).

- Associated features:
  - Premonitory symptoms and aura occur in migraine.
  - Photophobia, phonophobia and movement sensitivity are features of migraine
  - Autonomic features occur periorbitally in cluster headache.
  - Gastrointestinal disturbances are most commonly associated with migraine (but can occur with any headache).

- Precipitating or exacerbating factors:
  - Onset with exertion—SAH or benign exertional headache.
  - Hormone changes—pregnancy, menstruation, perimenopause. Particularly migraine. Combined oral contraception.
  - Lifestyle or environmental changes—stress, too much sleep, missing a meal, weather changes. Particularly migraine.
  - Substance triggers. Particularly migraine.
  - Stimulation of trigger points on face and mouth such as exposure to cold air or brushing teeth can provoke trigeminal neuralgia.
  - Changes in body position can intensify headache associated with nasal disease or CSF pressure.
  - Worse with coughing, sneezing on wakening—abnormalities of CSF pressure.

- Relieving factors:
  - Lying in a dark room helps to relieve migraine.
  - Pressure on trigger points can help migraine.
  - Vigorous movement, sitting upright, rocking can relieve cluster.
  - Tension type can be relieved by relaxation and rest or exercise.

- Social and employment history
  - Stressful life events can have a significant role in headache.
  - Alcohol, smoking, drugs or sexual activity may be relevant.
  - Heating at home, other family members—always think about carbon monoxide.
  - Explore potential work-related exposure to drugs or toxins.

- Sleep habits
  - Sleep apnoea can cause morning headache.
  - Hypnic headache wakes only from sleep.

- Family history
  - 60% of migraineurs have a parent and 80% a first-degree relative with migraine. A useful clue to support diagnosis.

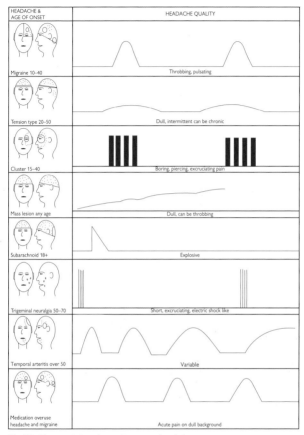

Fig. 1.2 Characteristics of some important headaches.

- Medication and past headache history
  - Treatment response can support a diagnosis
  - Often previous treatment failure as a result of inadequate dosing or continuation of drug.
  - Medication overuse headache may be a problem, particularly with over-the-counter medication.
  - Many patients will have tried complementary therapies.
- Medical history
  - Distal disease particularly tumour can present as headache
  - Depression and anxiety are co-morbid with migraine and can be a cause of tension-type headache.
  - Co-morbidity may direct treatment options particularly depression, asthma, hypertension and epilepsy.

Framing the question
- Answers may be influenced by preconceived notions.
- Be aware of non-verbal clues.
- Put questions in an experiential format. For example, not 'does noise bother you?' but 'do you have to turn down the TV during an attack?'
- Treat questionnaire diagnosis with caution.

Examination
The examination rarely adds to the diagnosis, but a secondary cause must always be excluded.
- A full neurological examination is rarely possible within the constraints of the consultation in primary care.
- Fundoscopy and blood pressure measurement are minimum requirements. (Although, with the exception of malignant hypertension, the relationship between blood pressure and headache is contested.)
- A simple proforma that would exclude most pathologies is suggested in Table 1.15.

Formulating a management plan
- Take patients' preferences into account,
- Provide supportive literature particularly for any drugs prescribed.
- Discuss implications for using unlicensed drugs (see Table 1.16).

Table 1.15 A simple examination proforma

- Pupillary responses and fundoscopy
- Visual fields
- Eye movements (superior, inferior, lateral)
- Facial movements (wrinkle forehead, grimace with teeth)
- Protrude tongue
- Outstretch arms, palms upwards for palmar drift
- With eyes closed, touch nose with finger (upper limb pyramidal, posterior column
- Finger dexterity (play piano)
- Rapid hand movement, tap fingers of one hand on opposite palm and vice versa (cerebella coordination)
- Limb and plantar reflexes
- Standing—feet together and eyes closed for balance (Romberg's test)
- Walk heel to toe along a straight line
- Walk on heels, walk on toes
- Check for trigger points particularly over occiput, posterior neck and upper shoulders
- Active neck movement (rotation, lateral flexion)
- In the acute setting, include temperature, rash, neck stiffness, temporal artery tenderness if over 50

Table 1.16 The use of licensed and unlicensed drugs

- Licensed drug
  - Licensed for use in migraine
  - Unlicensed for use but licensed in other areas, in accepted use for migraine and used 'off label', e.g. sodium valproate.
  - Unlicensed for migraine but licensed in other areas and used 'off label'. Not widely used in migraine, e.g. ACE inhibitors.
- Unlicensed drug
  - Available on prescription but no product licence, e.g. flunarizine.
  - Not available on prescription and no product licence.
- The prescriber accepts increasing clinical and product liability with descending order as above.
  - Providing the drug has a recognized clinical indication and was appropriately prescribed, clinical liability is defensible.
  - The prescriber's risk is for product liability if prescribing off licence
  - Benefits must be assessed against risks and liabilities with documented consent of the patient.

Using the headache consultation as a therapeutic intervention—neuro-linguistic programming

The therapeutic value of the physician–patient interaction has long been recognized. Neuro-linguistic programming (NLP) is a practical and eclectic approach which draws upon a number of techniques. It studies internal experience and how it can be changed. It makes no claim for a theoretical underpinning bur accommodates what works, and has a number of useful insights that are particularly relevant for headache.

The starting point is to recognize we all have are own map of the world. The map is never the territory but a representation of it. NLP is the art of changing these maps.

Overall ideas central to NLP

- *Neuro:* is about how we all experience the world through our senses, and do things internally with it to make our own experience unique. Most people appreciate this, but knowing *how* others experience the world can be very useful.
- *Linguistic:* we use words to describe our experience. The words we use are important and affect how we feel about the experience.
- *Program:* we tend to respond to certain stimuli in a predictable way. These thoughts and behaviours are also known as patterns or programs. If we know what these are and how we do them, we have a choice as to whether we follow a set pattern or change it.

Basic principles of NLP

- Rapport. For effective communication you need to meet another in their model of the world.
- Sensory awareness. An ability to pick up the cues patients give not only in what they say but in the body language and visual cues. Sensory awareness includes that to one's own responses also.
- Behavioural flexibility. To realize that we have choice in how we behave and to be able to make that choice will move things on much more quickly and in a better way than if there are a limited set of responses. This can succinctly be put as 'If what you are doing isn't working, do something different'.
- Outcome focus. It is useful to know what we are aiming for. What does the patient want? What does the physician want? It can be useful to set the intention at the start of the consultation. For example, the practitioner could start the consultation with 'I want to understand what your experience is like as a way to understand what is going on so that I can be useful to you', and at the end of the consultation ask, 'did I achieve my outcome; did the patient achieve theirs?'

Investigating the headache

Investigating the headache

Although headache diagnosis is based primarily on history supported by examination, further investigation may be indicated:
• To exclude a secondary underlying cause
• To reassure both patient and doctor
• For medical legal concerns
• To establish a baseline or contraindications for drug treatment

The decision to investigate will depend on:
• Whether the potential benefits outweigh the costs and disadvantages.
• The context of the consultation.
  • Patients seen in secondary care will often anticipate the exclusion of pathology and consultants will be under pressure to make a diagnosis at the first appointment.
  • In primary care, few patients will anticipate immediate investigation and the management focus is on careful follow-up.

Encephalography
• EEG is no longer recommended for the routine evaluation of patients with headache. However, it can be useful if:
  • Investigating associated symptoms suggestive of co-morbid seizures.
  • Alteration in consciousness.
  • Suspected encephalopathy.

Lumbar puncture
• Diagnosis of:
  • SAH
  • Meningitis or encephalitis
  • High or low CSF pressure
  • Inflammatory diseases, e.g. sarcodosis
  • Malignant infiltration (cytology)
• Myelography for leak localization in intracranial hypotension.
• Disadvantages
  • Post-lumbar puncture headache
  • Coning if pressure is high (a normal CT does not exclude high pressure)
• Contraindications (see Table 2.3)
  • Raised intracranial pressure
  • Local infection at LP site
  • Bleeding diathesis including anticoagulants

Table 2.1 Some terms used to define tests

- Sensitivity—percentage of individuals who have a disease and a positive test. A high sensitivity test will identify most people with the problem.
- Specificity—the percentage of patients who do not have the disease and have a negative test. If specificity is high there are few false positives.
- Positive predictive value. The proportion of patients with a positive test that are currently diagnosed.
- Negative predictive value. The proportion of patients with a negative test that are currently diagnosed.
- Likelihood ratio. How much more likely an event is in one population than another (likelihood ratio = post-tests odds/pre-test odds)

Table 2.2 Characteristics of normal CSF

- Clear, colourless
- Opening pressure 8–16mm
- Cells/µl <5 lymphocytes
- Protein 0.1–0.45g/l
- Glucose >50% blood glucose
- No xanthochromia

Blood tests

Rarely indicated in first presentation of headache, but useful if headache persists. May be indicated prior to starting medication. See Table 2.4.

Plain X-ray

Now superseded and rarely indicated. Useful for:
- Fracture
- Penetrating injuries
- Padget's disease

Computed tomography

- CT employs digital geometry processing to generate a 3-dimensional image from a large series of 2-dimensional X-rays taken around a single axis of rotation. Spiral rotation is also possible.
- Scanning is done with or without IV contrast.
- Thinner slices increased resolution. IV contrast enhancement can opacify blood vessels and identify blood–brain barrier breakdown due to tumour, infection, inflammation.
- Pregnancy is not a contraindication for CT of the head.
- Advantages
  - Less expensive than MRI
  - Higher sensitivity for SAH in first 3 days (see Table 2.5).
- Disadvantages
  - Radiation dose is ~70 times higher than a chest X-ray for a head CT.
  - Less sensitive than MRI. Can miss 10% of tumours.
  - Risks associated with contrast agents—potentially life threatening and include allergic reactions, kidney damage.

Magnetic resonance imaging

- MRI relies on the relaxation properties of hydrogen nuclei in water that have been excited in a magnetic field. As the nuclei relax they emit electromagnetic radiation in the radiofrequency range which is processed to generate an image. Contrast and properties of water are altered in disease states.
- Contrast agents can delineate areas of interest. Gadolinium provides high sensitivity for detection of vascular tissues and brain perfusion.
- Magnetic resonance angiography (MRA) intensifies blood flow non-invasively and has effectively replaced catheter angiography.
- Other approaches such as MRI spectroscopy and functional MRI are largely experimental.
- Advantages
  - Better resolution than CT except for early bleeds.
  - No known side effects with MRI. Safe in pregnancy (except 1st trimester).
- Disadvantages
  - Higher cost.
  - Metallic structures prevent use, e.g. aneurysm clips, pacemakers.
  - Claustrophobic—although improved on later models. 10% of patients affected

Table 2.3 Causes of high or low CSF pressure

Causes of increased CSF pressure	Causes of decreased CSF pressure
• Idiopathic intracranial hypertension	• Subarachnoid blockage
• Hydrocephalus	• Leakage of spinal fluid
• Subarachnoid haemorrhage	• Severe dehyrdration
• Meningitis	• Circulatory collapse
• Congestive heart failure	
• Cerebral oedema	

Table 2.4 Blood tests for headache

Primary investigations

- Full blood count—anaema, leukaemia and infection can cause headache.
- Thrombocytopenia
- ESR and CRP—can indicate temporal arteritis or systemic disease.
- Creatinine—renal failure can cause headache.
- Calcium—to exclude hypercalcaemia.
- Thyroid function test—headache can be associated with hypothyroidism.
- Liver function test—could indicate metastatic disease

Secondary investigations

- VDRL
- HIV
- Lyme antibodies
- Antinuclear antibodies, lupus anticoagulant, anticardiolipin antibodies

Ultrasonography

Mainly superseded by other techniques

- Carotid artery Doppler
  - Arterial dissection
  - ID of atheromatous plaque
- Transcranial Doppler

Uses temporal bone as acoustic window

  - Midline shift
  - Supratentorial haematomas, aneurysms, arteriovenous malformations (AVMs)

Table 2.5 Probability of recognizing haemorrhage on CT after the event

Time after event	Probability %
Day 0	95
Day 3	74
Week 1	50
Week 2	30
Week 3	Almost zero

Table 2.6 Sensitivity of CT and MRI

CT	MRI
• More accurate for haemorrhage early after event	• More sensitive than CT particularly for posterior fossa and cervicomedullary lesions
• Will miss ~10% of space-occupying lesions particularly in the posterior fossa	• More accurate than CT for • White matter abnormalities • Venous sinus thrombosis • Space-occupying lesions • Meningeal disease • Pituitary pathology

Who to investigate

Although there are many secondary causes of headache, this chapter focuses on the ever-present concern that headaches may be due to an underlying space-occupying lesion and in particular a brain tumour.

Background

- Gliomas are the most common primary tumours in adults (65% incidence).
  - They arise from the glial supporting cells of the CNS and are further divided as to their cell of origin, e.g. astrocytoma, oligodendroglioma.
  - The overall 5-year survival is 20%.
  - Incidence increases rapidly above the age of 50 (see Fig. 2.1)
- Meningiomas are usually benign and accessible to surgery (20% incidence). The 10-year survival is 80%. 5% are malignant.
- Other tumours arise from local cell types, e.g. pituitary tumours, acoustic neuromas.
- Rarer tumours include ependymomas, medulloblastomas and other primitive tumours, lymphomas and haematopoiedic tumours (<5% incidence),
- Secondary tumours are the most common cause of brain malignancy in adults.
  - 50% of cases result from primary bronchial carcinoma, with patients with small cell lung cancer being particularly susceptible.
  - 20% of cases result from breast cancer.
  - Patients with melanoma constitute >10% of cases, despite the relative rarity of this malignancy.
  - Other important primary sites are renal cell carcinoma, oesophageal and rectal cancers.
- Tissue diagnosis is often difficult and an alternative approach is to grade tumours according to their growth rate from high (Grade 4) to low (Grade 1).
- Other non-progressive space-occupying lesions such as cysts, AVMs and aneurysms occur with similar frequency to primary tumours but their contribution to headache is less certain (see Table 2.7).
- Risk factors for primary brain tumour are:
  - Gliomas occur more frequently in individuals with neurofibromatosis and tuberosclerosis.
  - A small percentage of patients have a recognizable hereditary disposition.
  - They can be induced by radiation, e,g, after therapeutic radiation.
  - Age.
  - Smoking and alcohol are not risk factors.

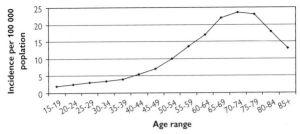

Fig. 2.1 Age-related rates per 100 000 population for malignant primary tumours.

Table 2.7 Results of imaging studies in a series of 1876 patients seen in secondary care with headache in the absence of any clinical findings

Diagnosis	Number
Cyst	3
Pituitary adenoma	3
Glioma	2
Meningioma	2
Hydrocephalus	2
Vascular malformation	2
Chiari malformation	1
CVA	1
Total number of patients	1876

(Source: Sempere A, *et al.* (2003). Neuroimaging in the evaluation of patients with non-acute headache. *Cephalalgia*. **25**: 30-5).

- The prevalence of headache and tumour is:
  - 70% of patients develop headache at some time during their illness.
  - Estimates of prevalence of headache at presentation are 23–56%.
  - Estimates of prevalence of isolated headache at presentation are 2–16%.

Risks of pathology with headache and no clinical signs

- Approximately 0.06% of a primary care population and 0.6% of a secondary care population presenting with headache and no clinical signs will have significant pathology (see Table 2.8).
- In a secondary care setting, the rates of significant findings on imaging in patients without neurological signs are:
  - Migraine—0.4% abnormalities
  - Tension-type headache—0.8% abnormalities
  - No formal diagnosis—3.7%

Advantages and disadvantages of imaging

The context in which the decision is made is important.

- Patients seen in secondary care will often anticipate the exclusion of secondary pathology and consultants will be under pressure to make a diagnosis at the first appointment.
- In primary care, few patients will anticipate further investigation, patients can be closely followed-up but doctors do experience difficulty diagnosing benign headaches.

Advantages

- Increase in quality and quantity of life. This will vary widely between types of lesion and in many cases may be marginal.
- Early prevention of distressing manifestations such as fitting may be important.
- Reassurance that no serious pathology is present. However, directly discussing a patient's concerns may reduce the need for unnecessary imaging.

Disadvantages

- The exposure of incidental pathology (0.6–2.8% of headaches screened) and the anxiety it incurs. There may also be implications for future life insurance applications.
- Potential distress caused by the investigation
- Inappropriate reassurance. CT is less sensitive than MRI and can overlook significant pathology
- The cost of investigation represents a missed opportunity of resources being utilized elsewhere

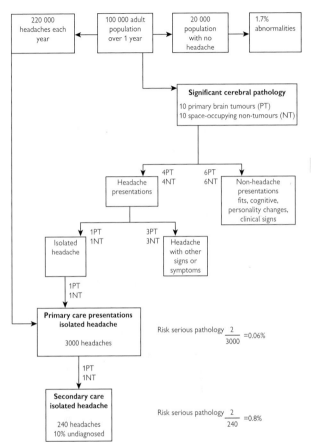

Fig. 2.2 Approximate top-down estimate of serious pathology and isolated headache in an adult population of 100 000 over a period of 1 year. Isolated headache caused by secondary tumour is excluded. PT= primary tumour, NT= space occupying lesion non-tumour.

Who should be imaged?

- The decision to investigate is based on a number of complex clinical, contextual and economic factors informed by a limited, poor quality evidence base. A useful guidance from the perspective of primary care is:

- **Red Flags**—presentations where the probability of an underlying tumour is likely to be >1%. These warrant urgent investigation.
  - Papilloedema.
  - Significant alterations in consciousness, memory, confusion or coordination.
  - New epileptic seizure,
  - New-onset cluster headache (non-urgent and include pituitary fossa views),
  - History of cancer elsewhere particularly breast and lung.
- **Orange Flags**—presentations where the probability of an underlying tumour is likely to be between 0.1 and 1%. These need careful monitoring and a low threshold for investigation.
  - New headache where a diagnosis has not emerged after 8 weeks from presentation.
  - Headache with abnormal findings on neurological examination or other neurological symptoms.
  - Headache aggravated by exertion or Valsalva manoeuvre.
  - Headaches associated with vomiting.
  - Headaches that have been present for some time but have changed significantly, particularly a rapid increase in frequency.
  - New headache in a patient over 50.
  - Headaches that wake patients from sleep.
  - Isolated confusion
- **Yellow Flags**—presentations where the probability of an underlying tumour is likely to be <0.1% but above the population rate of 0.01%. These need appropriate management, but the need for follow-up is not excluded.
  - Diagnosis of migraine or tension-type headache.
  - Weakness or motor loss.
  - Memory loss.
  - Personality change,

A common problem in primary care is isolated headache where a clear diagnosis is not obtained. Table 2.8 shows an approach to this problem.

Table 2.8 Guidance for headache in primary care without clinical signs where no diagnosis can be made

- At presentation
  - Exclude urgent headache (risk >1%).
  - Check blood pressure, fundoscopy and ESR if >50 years to exclude temporal arteritis.
  - If no diagnosis cannot be made tell patient—'*There is no evidence of anything serious underlying your headache but I would like to review you in 1 month*'.
  - Ask patient to keep a headache diary.
- At 1 month
  - Exclude urgent features.
  - Neurological examination, particularly cranial nerves.
  - Assess memory and cognitive function during interview.
  - Assess for symptoms that would indicate primary lesion elsewhere.
  - Consider blood screen to exclude systemic illness or evidence of primary tumour elsewhere—FBC, ESR, CRP, LFT, creatinine, electrolytes, glucose, thyroid function.
  - If diagnosis is still uncertain tell patient '*There is still no evidence of anything serious but I would like to review you again in another month*'.
- At 2 months
  - Exclude urgent features.
  - Examination as before.
  - If diagnosis is still uncertain tell patient '*There is still no evidence of anything serious underlying your headache but we need to discuss whether it would be appropriate to have a brain scan. Two in every 100 people like you will show an incidental finding that may give rise to unnecessary anxiety. This may have implications for future life insurance cover. 4 in every 100 people like you will show findings we may need to do something about*'.
  - MRI is the investigation of choice. If CT is the only practical option the patient should be cautioned that up to 10% of lesions can be missed.
  - Order blood investigations as above if not previously taken, in addition to test dependent on symptoms and history, e.g. VDRL, Lyme, antiphospholipids (see above)
- If patient and doctor decide against imaging, review again in 1 month. A normal investigation does not eliminate the need for further review and management of the headache.

Images of headache

Computed tomography

- CT scanning is most commonly requested in the acute setting. It readily illustrates intracranial haemorrhage, space-occupying lesions and hydrocephalus.
- It allows good demonstration of bony structures, and assessment of calcification within a lesion.
- IV contrast can be used to help characterize lesions on CT, or increase their conspicuity.
- CT angiography is excellent at identifying vascular abnormalities such as intracranial aneurysms, venous sinus thromboses and AVMs.
- On a practical level, CT is both widely available, and relatively quick.
  - These are important considerations for the unwell or agitated patient.
  - There is minimal enclosure of the head; so claustrophobic patients tend to cope reasonably well.
  - The short acquisition time required for the images minimizes movement artefact.
  - Monitoring unstable or anaesthetized patients is more straightforward in CT than in an MRI scanner.

Magnetic resonance imaging

- MRI has an important role in the imaging of headache, but is predominantly used as a secondary tool.
- This is largely due to more limited availability, and the length of time required to acquire images. The long scan time means that any movement, even that of deep breathing, produces artefact which severely affects the images produced.
- The main advantages of MRI over CT are improved contrast resolution, the ability to analyse the internal architecture of a lesion using different pulse sequences and the ability to acquire images in any plane.
  - MRI is the modality of choice for the evaluation of intra- and extra-axial tumours. It provides excellent views of the brainstem and pituitary, both of which are poorly seen with CT.
  - It allows the demonstration of white matter disease earlier and more clearly than with CT.
- Magnetic resonance angiography (MRA) and magnetic resonance venography (MRV) can be undertaken to illustrate AVMs, aneurysms and venous sinus thromboses. Gadolinium is the most commonly used contrast medium.
- Anyone entering the MRI scanner room must complete a safety questionnaire. The magnet is always on and is a significant hazard.
- The staff in an MRI unit are a good source of advice on the contraindications to MRI, as is the website www.mrisafety.com

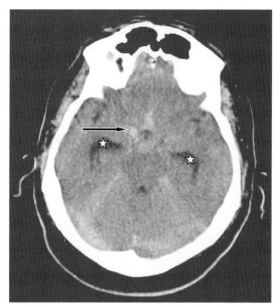

Fig. 2.3 Non-enhanced axial CT image.

Clinical scenario

A 45-year-old female presented to the Emergency Department with a thunderclap headache. She vomited three times and her GCS dropped from 15 to 13 (Fig. 2.3)

Diagnosis: SAH

- The most common cause of SAH is trauma.
- Around 85% of non-traumatic SAH is due to a ruptured aneurysm. The peak age is 40–60, SAH is more common in women.
- There is an increased risk with smoking and a family history of aneurysmal SAH.
- Non-enhanced CT (NECT) is the best imaging tool. If the CT is positive then a CT angiogram is acquired at the same sitting to detect aneurysms.
- NECT is positive in 95% in first 24h. By 1 week <50% are positive.

Images explained

Axial NECT demonstrates acute SAH. This is shown as high density in the basal cisterns (arrow). There is also early hydrocephalus as shown by the dilated temporal horns of the lateral ventricles.

Clinical scenario

A 30-year-old male presented with headache, intermittent nausea and vomiting (Figs 2.4 and 2.5)

Diagnosis: colloid cyst

- Almost all colloid cysts occur at the foramen of Munro. They measure up to 3cm and cause intermittent hydrocephalus by blocking drainage of CSF from the lateral ventricles.
- They most commonly present in the 3rd–4th decade with headache (60% of patients).
- On CT two-thirds of colloid cysts are hyperdense. On T1-weighted MRI two-thirds are of high signal and on T2-weighted MRI the majority are isointense to white matter.
- Colloid cysts do not enhance.
- The diagnosis can usually be made on either CT or MRI.

Images explained

On the NECT there is a hyperdense lesion in the anterosuperior roof of the 3rd ventricle (arrow). There is lateral splaying of the posterior part of the frontal horns of the lateral ventricle. The lesion is well shown on the coronal MRI (arrow). It is hyperintense to white matter.

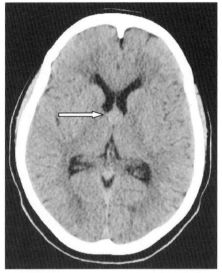

Fig. 2.4 Non-enhanced axial CT image.

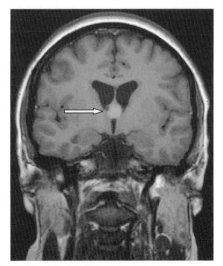

Fig. 2.5 Coronal T1-weighted image.

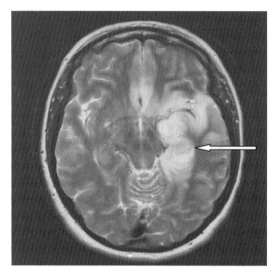

Fig. 2.6 T2-weighted axial MRI.

Clinical scenario

A 20-year-old male student presented to his GP with fever and headache. At the surgery, he suffered a seizure and was taken to the Emergency Department (Fig. 2.6).

Diagnosis: herpes simplex virus (HSV) encephalitis

- The highest incidence is in adolescents and young adults.
- Typically the temporal lobes and the cingulate gyrus are affected while the basal ganglia are spared. Usually there is bilateral but asymmetrical involvement.
- Patients present with fever, headache and seizures. Fewer than 30% of patients have an altered mental state or focal neurology.

Image explained

On the T2-weighted axial MRI images there is increased signal in the grey and subcortical white matter, primarily in the left medial temporal lobe (arrow). There is local mass effect as demonstrated by the effacement of the sulci.

Low attenuation and mass effect is rarely demonstrated in the first 3 days of the illness on NECT. On contrast-enhanced CT (CECT), HSV encephalitis classically demonstrates patchy gyriform enhancement of the temporal lobes, but this is a late finding. MRI is the preferred imaging modality. HSV encephalitis changes may be demonstrated within 2 days of onset. Affected regions typically demonstrate low signal on T1-weighted images and high signal on T2-weighted images.

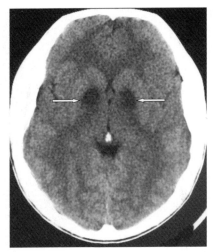

Fig. 2.7 Non-enhanced axial CT image.

Clinical scenario

A 75-year-old male presented with headache, nausea and vomiting. On examination he was found to have a gait disturbance and memory loss (Fig. 2.7).

Diagnosis: carbon monoxide poisoning

- Acute toxicity presents with a wide range of symptoms and signs, ranging from headache to confusion, coma and death.
- Mortality is increased if the patient is >75 years.
- Treatment is hyperbaric oxygen therapy.

Image explained

The globus pallidus is hypodense bilaterally (arrows). This is the most common finding in CO poisoning. Symmetrical hypodensity in the centrum semiovale and elsewhere in the deep cortical white matter is also recognized. These findings are not specific to CO poisoning, but are also seen in other causes of hypoxic brain injury. MRI is more sensitive than CT in detecting the effects of CO poisoning on the brain. T2-weighted images typically demonstrate high signal in the globus pallidus with a hypointense rim. There may also be confluent symmetric hyperintensity in the deep cortical white matter. Diffusion-weighted MRI is the best imaging modality for identifying lesions in the acute stage.

Clinical scenario

A 39-year-old male had a brief episode of loss of consciousness following a blow to the head. He regained consciousness and had no neurological deficit. However, 8h later he complained of headache and then dropped his GCS to 11/15 (Fig. 2.8).

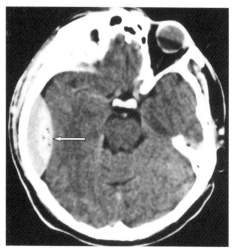

Fig. 2.8 Non-enhanced axial CT image.

Diagnosis: extradural haematoma (EDH)

- The most common cause of an EDH is trauma.
- 85% are associated with a skull fracture.
- 90% are due to arterial bleeding. Bilateral EDH or an EDH in the posterior fossa are associated with an increased mortality.
- The clinical impact and management of an EDH depend on its size and associated mass effect, as well as associated injuries.

Images explained

There is a right-sided EDH. The blood is trapped between the calvarium and outer dura. EDHs are usually lentiform in shape (arrow). They may cross dural attachments, but not suture lines. In this example, there is also air within the EDH due to the overlying fracture. The EDH is exerting local mass effect on the underlying brain.

Clinical scenario

A 27-year-old patient presented with headache, 3 weeks postpartum. On examination she was found to have papilloedema (Fig 2.9).

Diagnosis: venous sinus thrombosis

- There are a large number of predisposing factors, including pregnancy, the oral contraceptive pill, infection, trauma and coagulopathy.

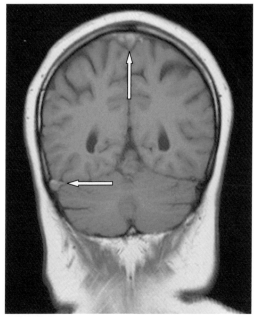

Fig. 2.9 Coronal T1-weighted MRI.

- Venous sinus thrombosis is more common in females.
- Clinical diagnosis can be difficult. Treatment is with anticoagulation.

Image explained

There is thrombosis evident in the superior sagittal sinus (vertical arrow) and right transverse sinus (horizontal arrow). Cerebral venous sinus thrombosis is well demonstrated on MRI as absence of flow void; the clot is hyperintense. The diagnosis can be confirmed with MRV.

On NECT the acute thrombus is of high attenuation. On CECT the 'empty delta sign' may be evident (non-enhancing thrombus at the torcula). CT venography demonstrates thrombus as a filling defect in the sinus.

Venous sinus thrombosis may be associated with venous infarction. This is often haemorrhagic.

Clinical scenario

A 15-year-old male presented with headache, vomiting and a visual field defect (Fig .2 10).

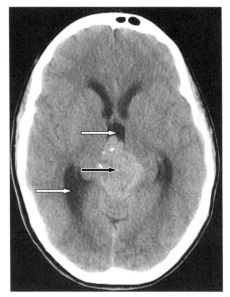

Fig. 2.10 Non-enhanced axial CT image.

Diagnosis: pineal tumour (pineoblastoma)
- Tumours in the pineal gland are uncommon in adults but account for up to 10% of brain tumours in the paediatric population.
- As pineal tumours often involve the adjacent ventricular system, they commonly present with the symptoms of hydrocephalus.
- If the tumours invade the tectal plate they may lead to an abducent nerve palsy and Parinaud syndrome.
- CSF seeding is common. Pineal tumours are usually germ cell tumours, and therefore α-fetoprotein or chorionic gonadotrophin are present in the CSF.
- Treatment is with surgical resection, radiation and chemotherapy.

Image explained
There is an irregular hyperdense mass arising from the pineal gland (black arrow). There is calcification within the lesion. It is causing hydrocephalus (white arrows). This is a typical appearance of a pineoblastoma.

On MRI T2-weighted images a pineoblastoma has a mixed signal, frequently demonstrating necrosis and haemorrhage. The calcification may not be as well appreciated on MRI. On T1-weighted images with IV contrast there is heterogeneous enhancement.

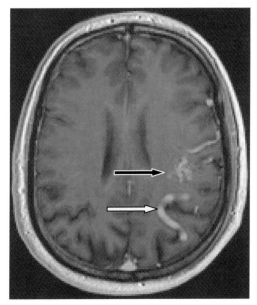

Fig. 2.11 Contrast-enhanced axial CT image.

Clinical scenario

A 24-year-old female presented with sudden onset of a severe headache (Fig. 2.11).

Diagnosis: arteriovenous malformation (AVM)

- The majority of AVMs cause symptoms.
- 50% will present with headache and haemorrhage. 25% present with a seizure.
- Patients with AVMs usually present between 20 and 40 years of age.
- The risk of haemorrhage increases with age. Treatment is with stereotactic radiosurgery, embolization or surgery.

Image explained

There is vivid enhancement of the AVM within the left cerebral hemisphere. The enlarged draining vein (white arrow) is particularly clearly seen leading away from the central nidus (black arrow). On a NECT, if the AVM is small it may not be demonstrated. 30% will show calcification. On unenhanced MRI images the signal varies with flow rates. Classically an AVM appears as a mass of flow voids that enhance avidly with contrast. Conventional cerebral angiography is necessary to demonstrate the 3 components of the AVM: the enlarged arteries, the central nidus and the draining vein.

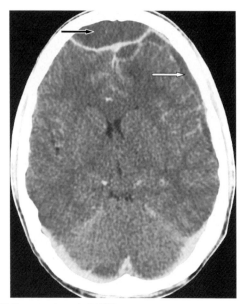

Fig. 2.12 Contrast-enhanced axial CT image.

Clinical scenario

A 36-year-old man presented with a chronic history of purulent nasal discharge and subacute headache (Fig. 2.12).

Diagnosis: extradural and subdural empyema secondary to sinusitis

- If the infection in sinusitis erodes through the bony walls of the sinuses it can spread to involve adjacent structures.
- The sequealae of sinusitis include orbital cellulitis and, as demonstrated here, intracranial abscess formation.

Image explained

There is a hypodense extradural collection anteriorly (black arrow). In addition, there is a second collection superficial to the left cerebral hemisphere in the subdural space (white arrow). The collections are causing mass effect with effacement of the cerebral sulci and distortion of the anterior horns of the lateral ventricles. Intracranial empyemas are demonstrated more clearly and earlier on MRI than on CT.

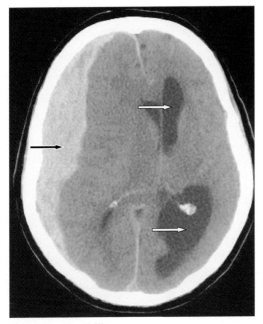

Fig. 2.13 Non-enhanced axial CT image.

Clinical scenario

A 24-year-old builder was brought to the emergency department having fallen 20ft from scaffolding. He had initially lost consciousness but then became lucid although complaining of headache (Fig. 2.13).

Diagnosis: acute subdural haematoma (SDH)

- Acute SDHs are commonly caused by trauma, as either a direct blow or a shearing force.
- There can be an associated skull fracture, as well as underlying brain injury.
- The insult causes rupture of the veins that traverse the subdural space.
- There is high morbidity with injuries of this nature.

Image explained

There is a large right-sided SDH (black arrow). As the blood is able to cross the cranial suture lines, SDHs tend to adopt a crescentric shape. A SDH cannot cross dural attachments. The high density of the blood indicates this is an acute haemorrhage. The pressure caused by the haematoma has led to a shift of the midline structures to the left. There is partial effacement of the right lateral ventricle, due to obstruction at foramen of munroe hydrocephalus of the left ventricular system (white arrows). Midline shift is a poor prognostic indicator.

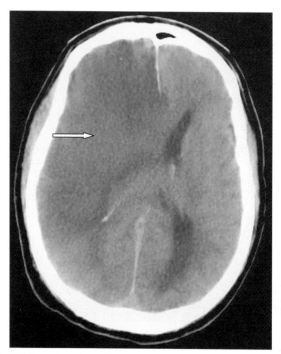

Fig. 2.14 Non-enhanced axial CT image.

Clinical scenario

A 90-year-old woman was found at home on the floor by her daughter. She was unable to move her left arm and leg. She had complained of a mild headache to her daughter the night before (Fig. 2.14).

Diagnosis: infarction in the territories of the right middle cerebral and anterior cerebral arteries

- CT is required in these patients to distinguish between ischaemic and haemorrhagic stroke, as well as to select patients for thrombolysis.
- MRI is usually reserved for patients with a negative CT, but is particularly useful in the posterior fossa where CT images are often degraded by streak artefact.

Image explained

There is a large hypodense area of brain parenchyma (arrow) in the territory supplied by the right internal middle and anterior cerebral arteries. There is involvement of both the grey and white matter, which is typical of an infarct. There is mass effect due to oedema, leading to shift of the midline structures to the left, and complete effacement of the right lateral ventricle.

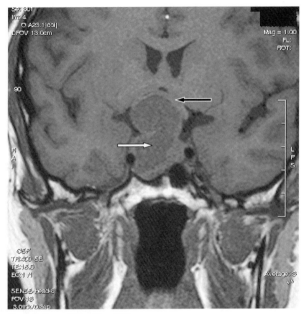

Fig. 2.15 Coronal T1-weighted MRI.

Clinical scenario

A 50-year-old woman was referred from her optician for investigation of visual field changes and headache. Having thought she needed new glasses, she was found to have a bitemporal hemianopia (Fig. 2.15).

Diagnosis: pituitary macroadenoma

- These non-malignant neoplasms originate in the pituitary fossa and can extend into adjacent areas.
- Extension superiorly into the suprasellar cistern, with subsequent compression of the optic chiasm, classically leads to a bitemporal hemianopia.
- Pituitary adenomas may be functional or non-functional; endocrine testing should be arranged.

Image explained

There is a low signal intensity mass arising from the pituitary fossa (white arrow) with superior extension into the suprasellar cistern. The optic chiasm is stretched over the tumour (black arrow). The pattern of enhancement is variable. Pituitary tumours can be difficult to identify on CT. MRI is the preferred imaging modality

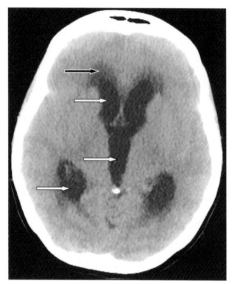

Fig. 2.16 Non-enhanced axial CT image.

Clinical scenario

A 22-year-old woman presented to her GP with a continuous headache not relieved by simple analgesia. Whilst awaiting further investigation, she was admitted to the Emergency Department with worsening of her headache and drowsiness (Fig. 2.16).

Diagnosis: hydrocephalus—due to congenital acqueduct stenosis

- Hydrocephalus can be caused by either obstruction to the flow of CSF, reduced absorption of CSF in the choroid plexus or excessive production by the arachnoid villi.
- Dilatation of the ventricles leads to compression of the brain parenchyma, causing symptoms of headache, irritability and drowsiness.
- Causes of obstructive hydrocephalus include aqueduct stenosis, tumour and a colloid cyst.
- Non-obstructive causes of hydrocephalus include SAH and meningitis.

Image explained

There is symmetrical enlargement of the lateral and third ventricles (white arrows) with low attenuation in the periventricular white matter due to trans-appendymal CSF flow (black arrow). The hydrocephalus is causing effacement of the cerebral sulci. Hydrocephalus is equally well demonstrated on CT and MRI, but an MRI is essential in the investigation of the cause hydrocephalus primarily to identify obstructing lesions, particularly in the posterior fossa.

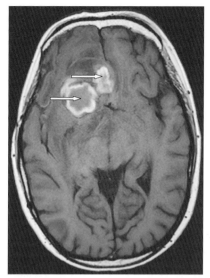

Fig. 2.17 Coronal T1-weighted MRI.

Clinical scenario

A 65-year-old male complained of increasing headache over several months associated with confusion (Fig. 2.17).

Diagnosis: right frontal glioblastoma multiforme (GBM)

- GBM are the most aggressive primary brain tumours.
- They are more common in males in the >65 age group and occur most commonly in the frontal and temporal lobes.
- Primary brain tumours do not metastasize outside the CNS, but may spread along white matter tracts and via the ventricular system or subarachnoid space.

Image explained

The post-contrast T1-weighted MRI demonstrates a large enhancing mass lesion in the right frontal region (arrows). The mass is surrounded by white matter (vasogenic) oedema and is causing local mass effect with efface-ment of the cerebral sulci, and shift of midline structures to the left.

Severe headache of sudden onset

Introduction

Sudden onset headache is a common problem and often the primary concern is to exclude a subarachnoid haemorrhage (SAH). This chapter considers SAH in detail and overviews other common causes of a sudden onset or 'thunderclap headache' (TCH).

The IHS definition of a primary TCH is a high-intensity headache of abrupt onset reaching maximal intensity in <1min, that does not recur regularly over subsequent months, and is not attributed to another disorder.

Subarachnoid haemorrhage

SAH should be considered in any patient presenting with sudden onset headache. Particularly significant is TCH type. The proportion of TCH caused by SAH varies from 11 to 25%, depending upon hospital or community setting.

- 80% of SAHs are caused by a ruptured intracranial aneurysm.
- Case fatality is ~50%, and one third of patients remain dependent.
- Patients sometimes give a history of a sudden, severe, headache lasting >1h, in the previous 4 weeks. This has been termed a 'sentinel' headache. However, some 'sentinel' headaches may actually represent small SAHs that did not receive correct or timely investigation; the term is therefore misleading and arguably should be abandoned.

Presentation

- When a cerebral aneurysm ruptures, blood is forced under high pressure into the subarachnoid space.
- Classically patients present with a sudden onset severe headache of a thunderclap nature. Consciousness may be impaired or lost. Rarely, consciousness is lost without any preceding complaint.
- The headache may be followed by nausea, vomiting, neck stiffness or photophobia. There may be a mild fever.
- Seizures occur in 10–25% of cases.
- Lateralizing focal neurological signs are absent in the majority of cases, although if present they can indicate the site of the aneurysm (e.g. an ipsilateral pupil involving third nerve palsy in a posterior communicating artery aneurysm). Rarely blood can rupture into adjacent brain or clot in the insular cistern and produce focal neurological signs.

Investigations

- Blood investigations
  - Full blood count. White cell count to help with differential diagnoses and haemoglobin because a significant anaemia can potentially affect the sensitivity of the CT.
  - Coagulation studies to exclude a coagulopathy.
  - Electrolytes—low sodium can occur secondary to cerebral salt wasting.

Table 3.1 Causes of thunderclap headache

- Subarachnoid haemorrhage
- Other vascular causes
  - Cerebral venous thrombosis
  - Arterial dissection, e.g. vertebral/carotid artery dissection
  - Ischaemic and haemorrhagic stroke
  - Intracerebral, intraventricular, extradural, or subdural haemorrhage;
  - Vasculitides
  - Reversible cerebral vasoconstriction syndrome (RSVS)
- Non-vascular causes
  - Spontaneous intracranial hypotension
  - Hypertensive encephalopathy
  - Arnold–Chiari malformation
  - Pituitary apoplexy
  - 3rd ventricle colloid cysts
  - Intracranial infection
  - Acute hydrocephalus
  - Space-occupying lesions
  - Other non-neurological conditions such as acute sinusitis and glaucoma
    can also cause relatively abrupt onset pain.
- Primary headaches (a diagnosis of exclusion)
  - Primary cough, coital and exertional headache
  - Primary thunder clap headache
  - Migraine
  - Cluster headache

Table 3.2 Causes of subarachnoid haemorrhage

- Aneurysmal—80%
- Non-aneurysmal—20%

Of these:
- 2/3rds perimesencephalic
- The remainder
  - Arterial dissection
  - AVM
  - Vascular lesions of spinal cord
  - Septic aneurysm
  - Pituitary apoplexy
  - Drugs
  - Trauma

- Magnesium—low magnesium associated with poor outcome,
- Glucose—low glucose is associated with poor outcome,
- Electrocardiogram (ECG)—cardiac arrhythmias may occur in SAH
- Radiological investigations
  - Non-contrast CT performed early (<24h) has a sensitivity of up to 98% within 12h and 93% within 24h for detection of blood.
  - Beyond 24h the sensitivity of CT drops significantly.
  - Blood is frequently reabsorbed within 10–14 days.
  - Scans should be reviewed by an experienced radiologist.
- Lumbar puncture
  - If the CT scan does not identify a significant abnormality but SAH is suspected, an LP should be performed.
  - The primary reason is to examine for the presence of blood breakdown products (bilirubin and oxyhaemoglobin) using spectophotometry.
  - Four consecutive samples should be taken. The final CSF sample should be the one sent for spectrophotometry.
  - Following a haemorrhage into the CSF, red blood cells undergo lysis and phagocytosis. The liberated oxyhaemoglobin is converted *in vivo* in a time-dependent manner into bilirubin which, after centrifugation, produces a yellow pigment called xanthochromia. Oxyhaemoglobin may very unusually be found on its own after a SAH, but is much more likely to represent a traumatic tap.
  - Examination of the CSF using spectrophotometry to look for specific absorbance peaks is considered more accurate than looking at the sample with the naked eye for a yellow discoloration.
  - Other CSF constituents of protein, glucose, red and white cells should be examined. Serum glucose and serum bilirubin should also be tested.
- Subsequent investigations to identify the cause of a SAH
  - If a SAH is identified on the CT scan then it is necessary to identify the point of bleeding.
  - This is a cerebral aneurysm in 80% of cases. Table 3.2 outlines the causes of SAH.
  - Direct catheter angiography remains the gold standard, although centres are increasingly using non-invasive techniques such as CT angiography or MRA which allow 3-D reconstruction.
  - The sensitivity of CT angiography varies according to the diameter of aneurysm and reconstruction method, but is ~96% for aneurysms >3mm.

Complications of SAH

- Rebleeding
- Immediate cerebral ischaemia
- Delayed cerebral ischaemia—main period of risk between day 4 and 14, and due to vasospasm
- Hydrocephalus
- Fits

Table 3.3 Practical considerations of lumbar puncture

- It is frequently taught that the CSF bilirubin is a reliable test for a SAH if performed between 12h and up to 2 weeks after the bleed. Although the evidence base for these statements is relatively weak, guidelines often consider a delay of up to 12h advisable before performing the LP. Detection of CSF bilirubin declines over time. It is detected in 70% of cases after 3 weeks and in 40% after 4 weeks.

- The CSF opening pressure should always be recorded. May be elevated in SAH, but also in cerebral venous sinus thrombosis, intracranial infections and other causes of intracerebral insult. A low opening pressure may indicate spontaneous intracranial hypotension.

- A high serum bilirubin can spill over into in the CSF and thus result in a raised CSF bilirubin. It is therefore important to check serum bilirubin when performing the LP.

- Red blood cell lysis and thus *in vitro* formation of oxyhaemoglobin is exacerbated by vacuum transport systems. Light can cause the decay and destruction of bilirubin in a collected CSF sample. Vacuum transport systems should be avoided and CSF samples should be protected from light. The samples should be sent to the laboratory urgently to be centrifuged and examined.

- Cardiac arrhythmia or pulmonary oedema
- Hyponatraemia or hypomagnesaemia

Management of SAH

- Urgent advice from neurosurgeons and probable transfer to a neurosurgical unit
- Medical management
  - Nimodipine (oral) 60mg every 4h for 3 weeks to reduce cerebral vasospasm and reduce risk of poor outcome by ~5% (absolute risk reduction).
  - Ensure adequate hydration and treatment of low sodium (if present).
  - DVT prophylaxis with compression stockings.
  - Careful monitoring of vital signs, cardiac monitoring for arrythmia and regular recording of GCS.
- Occlusion of cerebral aneurysm. Neuroradiological guided endovascular occlusion as soon as possible with detachable metallic inert coils is generally used in preference to neurosurgical clipping unless there are technical reasons why coiling is not possible.

Table 3.4 Reasons for 'missing' a SAH

'Missed' SAH is a relatively frequent cause of medico-legal action in neurology. This may be due to:

- Failure to understand the spectrum of presentation of SAH headache. Typically SAH presents with sudden onset headache in the occipital region. However, proven SAH can present with headache evolving over minutes.
- Failure to understand the limitations of imaging, e.g. the 'drop off' in sensitivity of the CT scan over time. A restless patient may move in the scanner, resulting in images that are difficult to interpret.
- Failure to perform the LP/interpret the results appropriately
- Other symptoms may appear to prevail over the headache. Fits occur in 6–16% of patients with SAH at presentation, and management may focus on termination of the seizures without carefully considering the possible cause
- A SAH may cause a patient to lose consciousness and injure themselves through a fall or losing control of a vehicle. The clinical focus may then be directed towards management of the trauma without necessarily considering the cause. In such circumstances, even if blood is seen on a CT scan, this may be inappropriately attributed to trauma.

Cerebral venous thrombosis (CVT)

(See also Chapter 13)
- Although the predominant mode of onset in is gradual, 2–10% of CVT have a TCH presentation. Suspicion may arise from the history, imaging appearances and LP.
- Where CVT is suspected, specialist neuroradiological advice should be sought. Unenhanced CT may be normal in 25% of CVT. Abnormalities include venous infarction (often haemorrhagic), oedema or hyperintensity within a sinus, and can often be subtle. MRV is evolving as the non-invasive investigation imaging of choice.
- Abnormalities on LP are present in 50% of cases, comprising high red cell count, raised protein, raised opening pressure or a lymphocytosis.
- Secondary causes of CVT should always be considered.

Cervical arterial dissection

- Dissection of the carotid or vertebral arteries can cause headache and even SAH.
- It often follows a potentially traumatic event, but this can be minor (e.g. straining, coughing, hairwashing, chiropractor manipulation).
- Risk factors include Ehlers–Danlos syndrome, Marfan syndrome, α-1-antitrypsin deficiency and fibromuscular dysplasia.

Presentation
- Typically unilateral headache associated with an ipsilateral Horners syndrome, or with a unilateral headache and delayed focal cerebral ischaemic symptoms.
- Dissection of the vertebral arteries is less common than dissection of the carotid artery. Patients often have persistent occipitonuchal pain and are likely to have symptoms and signs of brainstem ischaemia.

Investigations
- CT or MRI of the brain will often show ischaemic changes in the relevant arterial territory of the dissection. MRI is significantly more sensitive than CT for the brainstem/posterior territory changes frequently found in vertebral dissections. Axial slices may demonstrate the dissected vessel, e.g. the 'doughnut' sign in carotid dissection.
- In most cases, ultrasound can detect carotid artery dissection. However, ultrasound is relatively user dependent, and suspicion of dissection requires confirmation.
- It is common practice to confirm the diagnosis with CT angiography or MRA. These are performed at the same time as the standard CT or MRI sequences.

Treatment
Historically, patients have been formally anticoagulated for a period of ~3–6 months, in part to prevent cerebral ischaemia from distal embolization. However, there is no conclusive evidence to demonstrate such an approach is superior to aspirin. In view of this, many physicians are therefore tending to avoid anticoagulation, and in preference prescribe antiplatelet agents.

Reversible segmental vasoconstriction syndrome (RSVS)

- RSVS is characterized by sudden onset of TCH and focal neurological deficits.
- It is due to reversible segmental cerebral vasoconstriction frequently associated with focal cerebral ischaemia.
- It may cause diagnostic confusion with primary angiits of the CNS.
- RSVS has been associated with several conditions, including pregnancy and puerperium ('postpartum angiopathy'), and use of vasoconstrictive medications.
- There is weak evidence to suggest that calcium channel inhibitors may be an effective therapy.

Spontaneous intracranial hypotension

(See also Chapter 11)
- Although the headache may be of sudden onset, it has an orthostatic component. When taking a history from a patient with acute headache it is important to question directly for the presence of postural symptoms
- Investigations will often facilitate diagnosis of this condition.
- The most consistent radiological changes are found on MRI.
  - Pachymeningeal enhancement with contrast
  - Posterior fossa crowding
  - Cerebellar tonsillar and chiasmal descent
  - Subdural collections.
- CSF (if performed) generally shows a low opening pressure with normal constituents.
- Further detection of leak (and the site of leakage) by means of cisternography or myelography is performed in tertiary centres.

Pituitary apoplexy

- Pituitary apoplexy is characterized by a sudden onset of headache (often retro-orbital), visual symptoms (altered acuity, visual field impairment, ocular motility problems), altered mental status, vomiting and hormonal dysfunction (e.g. hypopituitarism).
- It is generally caused by acute haemorrhage or infarction of the pituitary gland. An existing pituitary adenoma is usually present.
- The cause of the headache is uncertain but may be due to stretching of the dura in the walls of the sella supplied by meningeal branches of the trigeminal nerve or direct irritation of the trigeminal nerve.
- MRI, with pituitary cuts, electrolytes, glucose, pituitary hormone levels and visual field monitoring are required.
- Treatment consists of medical resuscitation, high dose corticosteroids, appropriate hormone replacement and evacuation of tumour if present.

Other acute headache dealt with elsewhere

- Primary cough, exertional and sex headache (See Chapter 12)
- Intracranial infection (See Chapter 13)
- Primary headache

The migraine attack

Epidemiology of migraine

The results of epidemiological studies vary according to methodology, setting and diagnostic criteria used.

The prevalence of migraine (number of cases in the population in a 1-year period)

Table 4.1 shows some global estimates of prevalence.
  Figure 4.1 shows the prevalence of migraine by age
- In the UK and USA, 15% of females and 6% of males suffer from migraine
- The prevalence of migraine is highest from ages 25 to 55 for both sexes at the time of peak economic productivity
- The prevalence of migraine decreases rapidly after the age of 55, particularly in females
- The relationship between migraine and socio-economic status is unclear, but evidence suggests an inverse relationship
- In the USA and western Europe, prevalence is higher in Caucasians than other races

The incidence of migraine (number of new cases occurring each year)

Figure 4.2 shows the incidence of migraine by age and sex.
- Incidence is maximal during adolescence
- Migraine begins earlier in males than in females
- Migraine with aura begins earlier than migraine without aura

The frequency of attacks in migraine sufferers

Number of attacks per month	%
1 or less	22%
2	22%
3	16%
4	15%
5 or more	25%

Table 4.1 Some global population estimates of migraine prevalence

Country	Males %	Females %
Europe and USA	6	15
Central and South America	6	15
Turkey	10	22
Asia	3	10
Africa	3	7

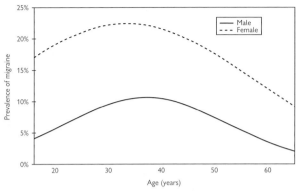

Fig. 4.1 The prevalence of migraine in England with age (data from Steiner T, *et al.* (2003). The prevalence and disability burden of adult migraine in England and their relationships to age, gender and ethnicity. *Cephalalgia.* **23** (7): 519-272).

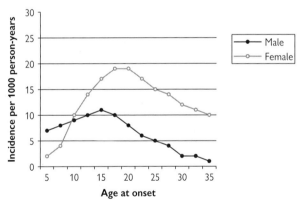

Fig. 4.2 The incidence of migraine with age and sex (data from Stewart W, *et al.* (1991). Age and sex specific incidence rates of migraine with and without visual aura. *Am J Epidemiol.* **134**: 1111-1120).

Making the diagnosis of migraine

IHS classifications are shown in Table 4.2. Migraine without aura is the most common:

A. At least 5 attacks fulfilling criteria B–D
B. Headache attacks lasting 4–72h (untreated or unsuccessfully treated)
C. Headache has at least two of the following characteristics:
  - Unilateral location
  - Pulsating quality
  - Moderate or severe pain intensity
  - Aggravating or causing avoidance of routine physical activity
D. During headache, at least one of the following:
  - Nausea and or vomiting
  - Photophobia and phonophobia
E. Not attributed to other disorder (a formal diagnosis of migraine therefore must include an examination to exclude another disorder).

The two major divisions are:
- Migraine without aura (previously known as common migraine)
- Migraine with aura (previously known as classical migraine); 20% of migraineurs

An aura is recurrent reversible focal neurological symptom that gradually develops over 5–20min and lasts for <60min.

Probable migraine is diagnosed when one criterion is absent.

From a practical perspective, the IHS criteria for diagnosis can be relaxed. Some sets of criteria that are found to be of high sensitivity for clinical use include:
- High disability, nausea, sensitivity to light.
- Nausea, photophobia, pain worse with exertion.
- Nausea, phonophobia, pulsating headache.
- Recurrent headaches that interfere with work, family or social function, lasting at least 4h, with no new or different headaches in past 6 months.
- A synthesis of available data is shown in Table 4.3

Some practical diagnostic pointers for migraine

- A family history of migraine increases the likelihood of a positive diagnosis
- Migraine is the most common headache presentation in primary and secondary care
- Headache that started in childhood is likely to be migraine
- Watch out for aura without headache
- Neck and tension-type headache in a migraine sufferer is likely to be part of the migraine spectrum

Table 4.2 IHS classification of migraine

1.1 Migraine without aura
1.2 Migraine with aura
    1.2.1 Typical aura with non-migraine headache
    1.2.2 Typical aura without headache
    1.2.3 Familial hemiplegic migraine (FHM)
    1.2.4 Sporadic hemiplegic migraine
    1.2.5 Basilar-type migraine
1.3 Childhood periodic syndromes that are commonly precursors of migraine
    1.3.1 Cyclical vomiting
    1.3.2 Abdominal migraine
    1.3.3 Benign paroxysmal vertigo of childhood
1.4 Retinal migraine
1.5 Complications of migraine
    1.5.1 Chronic migraine
    1.5.2 Status migrainosus
    1.5.3 Persistent aura without infarction
    1.5.4 Migrainous infarction
    1.5.5 Migraine-triggered seizure
1.6 Probable migraine
    1.6.1 Probable migraine without aura
    1.6.2 Probable migraine with aura
    1.6.3 Probable chronic migraine

Table 4.3 Approaches to migraine diagnosis

Positive likelihood ratios for the features: pulsatile quality of headache, duration of 4–72h, unilateral location, nausea or vomiting, disabling intensity:

- 24 (CI 1.5–388) for four or more features.
- 3.5 (CI 1.3–9.2) for three features.
- 0.41 (CI 0.32–0.52) for one or two features.

Co-morbidity and associations

Co-morbidity is a coincidental association of two conditions greater than chance. It heightens the index of suspicion for other relevant illnesses and may have implications for treatment options either by creating therapeutic opportunities or by imposing therapeutic limitations. Co-morbidity may be due to:

• Shared genetic or environmental factors
• Causal relationship between two conditions

Migraine and epilepsy

Epilepsy prevalence in migraineurs is 6% compared with a population prevalence of 0.5%. Care should be taken with drugs that lower convulsive thresholds such as TCAs and SSRIs when epilepsy is co-morbid. Rarely migraine can trigger a fit in a susceptible individual.

Migraine and psychiatric disease

There is an increased incidence in migraine sufferers of

• Depression
• Bipolar disorders
• Anxiety disorders
• Increased suicide attempts and ideation

Personality characteristics

Although there are many methodological problems, it has been suggested that migraineurs are more detailed, perfectionists and have more difficulties with relationships.

Vertigo

Vertigo is a vestibular symptom of abnormal motion

• Vertigo as a migrainous symptom (migrainous vertigo)
  • Benign paroxysmal positional vertigo (BPPV) of childhood is an early manifestation (2.8%)
  • Can occur in the absence of headache
  • Spontaneous or positional
  • Can last up to several days
  • Can be an aura symptom of basilar migraine <60min
• Vertigo syndromes that show an association with migraine
  • Meniere's disease
  • Benign paroxysmal vertigo
  • Motion sickness

Dizziness

Dizziness is a non-vestibular symptom of light headedness, unsteadiness or impending faint.

• Dizziness shows an association with migraine
• Orthostatic hypotension
• Co-morbid anxiety
• Antimigraine medication

Migraine and stroke

Migraineurs with aura have an increased relative risk compared with non-migraine sufferers. Possibilities are:

- Migrainous infarction. This is an infarct associated with an aura symptom in a similar territory demonstrated by neuroimaging, i.e migraine induces stroke (see later).
- Stroke-induced migraine (7% of strokes are silent).
  - Headache may occur as a symptom of ischaemic stroke or a TIA in 15–65% of patients (average 30%)
  - More likely if affecting the verterobasilar arterial territory and may be migraine like
  - Ischaemia-induced symptomatic migraine may be more common than migraine-induced ischaemic stroke
- Co-morbidities. There are a number of conditions that may give rise to migraine and stroke (e.g. CADASIL, AVMs, tumours, SAH, occipital epilepsy, basilar artery dissection, patent foramen ovale).
- Migraine may occur as a consequence of conditions that predispose to stroke (e.g. an underlying cerebral ischaemia provokes migraine).
- Migraine treatment may be causal, e.g vasoconstrictor drugs.
- Specific risk factors are
  - Migraine with aura
  - Onset of migraine with aura
  - Migraine duration >12 years
  - Attack frequency >12 years
- The association of migraine without aura as a risk factor for stroke is less clear.
- A meta-analysis of available studies has shown relative risks of:

Migraine in general	2.16 (95% CI 1.89–2.48)
Migraine with aura	2.88 (95% CI 1.89–4.39)
Women under 45	2.76 (95% CI 2.17–3.52)
Migraine without aura	1.56 (95% CI 1.03–2.36)

- The increased risk of migraine with aura and ischaemic stroke is further increased by smoking and use of the combined oestrogen–progesterone contraceptive pill:

Smoking	10.2 (95% CI 3.5-29.9)
Oral contraceptives	13.9 (95% CI 5.5–35.1)
Smoking + oral contraceptives	34.4 (95% CI 32.7–36.1)

White matter changes

Although studies are conflicting, there appears to be an increase in MRI-detected white matter abnormalities and silent cerebellar infarcts in subjects with migraine compared with those without. The relevance of these findings is currently not known.

Practical approaches to migraine and stroke

- The overall risk of stroke is small and the relative risk reduces with age
- Patients without aura can be reassured
- Co-morbid risk factors such as smoking, blood pressure, cholesterol, coagulation disorders, cardiac abnormalities may be additive. Lifestyle advice and risk factor management is appropriate.
- It is not know whether the demonstration of MRI white matter abnormalities in migraineurs is a risk factor for stroke
- Avoid oestrogen-containing oral contraceptives in women with aura

The migraine attack

Migraine pathophysiology

- A substantially inherited disorder.
- Fundamentally a disorder of the CNS.
- Vascular change in migraine is an epiphenomenon. The term 'vascular' is no longer appropriate in the context of migraine.
- Migraine involves activation of brain areas involved in the modulation of sensory input, especially in the brainstem.
- Familial hemiplegic migraine is an autosomal dominant disorder where ion channel dysfunction is the cause of the problem

The typical migraine attack is characterized by a number of phases which may or may not be recognized.

The premonitory phase

- Occurs in up to 60% of migraineurs
- Can occur up to 48h before an attack
- Symptoms include:
  - Psychological—depression, euphoria, irritability, restlessness, cognitive impairment, hyperactivity, fatigue, drowsiness.
  - Neurological—hyperosmia, photophobia, phonophobia.
  - General symptoms—disorders of taste, increased thirst, increased urination, anorexia, diarrhoea, food cravings, fluid retention.
- Useful from a management perspective as can trigger early treatment options.

The aura

- What is an aura? See Table 4.4.
- Visual aura is the most common. They can migrate across the visual field, rotate, oscillate or flicker, and be of varying colours and brightness There are a number of variations the most common being:
  - Scotoma
  - Simple flashes (photopsin), shimmer or jitter across visual field
  - Fortification spectrum
- Paraesthesia—these are the second most common aura occurring in ~30% of migraine with aura.
  - Usually starts in the hands and migrates up the arm
  - Can involve the face, lips and tongue
  - Is often followed by numbness
  - Is bilateral or becomes bilateral in half of patients
  - Can follow a visual aura
- Motor symptoms—occur in up to 18% of patients with aura such as weakness, ataxia, language disorders (dysarthria or aphasia).
- Delusions and disturbed consciousness such as deja vu, trance-like states, hallucinations.
- Visual distortions (Alice in Wonderland syndrome).
- Complex auras involving more than one symptom. Demand a high degree of suspicion for other conditions that include seizure, structural brain disease, cerebral vascular disease and primary psychiatric disorders.

Table 4.4 What is an aura?

- A reversible motor, sensory or other neurological symptom that is recurrent or stereotyped.
- Occur in 15–20% of patients, developing gradually over 5–20min and lasting usually <60min.
- Characterized by evolution of symptom.
- Can be simple (positive or negative) or complex.
- Can involve cortex or brainstem. The pathophysiological relationship with the mid brain 'migraine centre' is poorly understood.
- Is associated with headache (not necessarily migraine).
- Usually precedes the headache but can occur with it or in its absence.
- Neuroimaging fails to demonstrate an alternative explanation

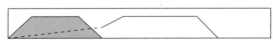

Fig. 4.3 The migraine headache.

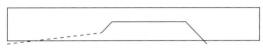

Fig. 4.4 The migraine premonitory phase.

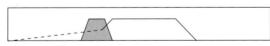

Fig. 4.5 The migraine aura.

- Migraine aura can occur without headache. The prevalence in the population may be as high as 1%. Differential diagnosis is TIA and focal seizures. TIA will come on suddenly, unlike an aura that will build up gradually.

The headache

- Headache is the cardinal feature of migraine
- Often pulsatile or throbbing and moderate to marked in severity
- Onset usually gradual with a range between 4 and 72h (shorter in children)
- Unilateral in 60% of cases and consistently occurs on the same side in 20%
- Pain can move from one side of the head to the other and radiate into the neck
- Scalp tenderness or allodynia can occur
- The headache can build up gradually over many hours. This can have the character of a tension-type headache. Patients can be unsure whether this headache will develop into a full-blown attack and when to use relevant therapy.

Between the attacks can experience idiopathic stabbing headache in 40% of patients. Described as 'ice pick' or 'jabs' or 'jolts'

Associated symptoms

- Associated phenomena often contribute to migraine-related disability, and vomiting can be more distressing than pain.
- Gastrointestinal disturbances are most common. This contributes to poor oral medication absorption.
  - Nausea occurs in 90% of patients
  - Vomiting occurs in 30% of patients
  - Anorexia and food cravings can occur
  - Diarrhoea occurs in 16% of patients
- Enhanced sensory perception or sensitivity
  - Photophobia
  - Phonophobia
  - Osmophobia
- Cognitive mood and cognitive changes
- Other associations include blurring vision, nasal stuffiness, sweating, flushing, fluid retention.

Postdrome

- Depressant effects—impaired concentration, lethargy, irritability, tiredness.
- Elevating effects—euphoria, heightened energy, heightened state of alertness

Table 4.5 Classification of auras

Typical auras	Atypical auras
Visual	*Primary sensory*
Simple—positive or negative	Olfactory
Complex, e.g. visual distortions	Auditory
Somaesthetic	Visceral
Simple—positive, e.g. tingling, negative e.g. numbness	Kinaesthetic
	Vestibulocochlear
Complex—somaesthetic distortions	Vertigo
Aphasic	Deafness
Expressive dysphasia	Drop attacks
Receptive dysphasia	*Motor*
Dyslexia	Chorea
	Dystonia
	Hemiplegia
	Higher integrative functions
	Memory
	Mood
	Perception and planning

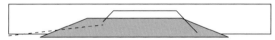

Fig. 4.6 Associated symptoms.

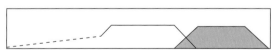

Fig. 4.7 The migraine postdrome.

Migraine variants and complications

The IHS classification of headache (ICHD-II) identifies several phenotypic variants of migraine (see Table 4.6). In addition, variants that are not recognized are described and complications (see Table 4.7).

- Individuals may experience several variants of migraine in their lifetime.
- The IHS criteria (ICHD-II) are not inclusive but serve as a framework not only to allow clinical characterization of migraine phenotypes but also to allow scientific study of the migraine variants.
- Their rigidity poses limitations if they are too strictly applied in clinical practice, but awareness of their core features allows recognition of the more common migraine variants.
- ICHD-II also includes a category of 'probable migraine' where some of the features suggestive of migraine are not apparent. The term 'migrainous' has been used previously. Often such individuals also have attacks of typical migraine.

Migraine without aura (MO)

- Previously referred to as 'common migraine,' attacks of MO are experienced by up to 80% of migraine sufferers.
- Cranial autonomic symptoms, such as lacrimation, conjunctival injection or nasal symptoms, are experienced by up to 50%.

Migraine with aura (MA)

- Previously referred to as 'classical migraine'.
- Attacks of headache associated with *transient, gradual onset, reversible* focal neurological symptoms. Experienced by up to 30% of migraine sufferers, and typical aura usually precedes or accompanies the migraine headache phase.
- Attacks may vary during a lifetime.
- Typically lasts 5–20min, with visual aura most common (reported by 95% of aura sufferers).
- Sensory symptoms and dysphasia are less common.
- Less commonly aura can manifest as other reversible neurological symptoms of dysfunction of other brain areas, e.g. the brainstem and other cortical areas.
- Aura is thought to be caused by a spreading wave of neuronal dysfunction termed cortical spreading depression, and not ischaemia. This, in combination with changes in central neurotransmitters and secondary effects on vascular tone and metabolic function, is a likely cause of symptoms.
- Triptans are ineffective in the aura phase of migraine in all types of aura.

Table 4.6 ICHD-II (adapted) migraine variant subtypes

- Migraine without aura (MO)
- Migraine with aura (MA)
  - Typical aura with migraine headache
  - Aura without headache (A)
  - Hemiplegic migraine (familial (FHM) and sporadic (SHM))
  - Basilar-type migraine
  - Retinal migraine
- Complications of migraine
  - Chronic migraine (CM)
  - Status migrainosus
  - Persistent aura without infarction
  - Migrainous infarction
  - Migraine-triggered seizures
- Childhood periodic syndromes that may herald later life migraine
  - Cyclic vomiting
  - Abdominal migraine
  - Benign paroxysmal vertigo of childhood

Table 4.7 Other migraine variants not described in ICHD-II

- Vestibular migraine
- Benign paroxysmal torticollis (of infancy)
- Alice in Wonderland syndrome
- Confusional migraine
- Migraine equivalents (aura without headache)
- Migraine aura status
- Menstrual migraine

Table 4.8 The characteristics of typical aura

- Evolves gradually over several minutes (in contrast to abrupt-onset TIAs), changing in size/location or on one side of the body, e.g. face to hand or vice versa.
- Manifests as fully reversible visual, sensory or speech symptoms either in isolation or sequentially in any combination.
- Typical visual aura is binocular, e.g. as homonymous spreading positive symptoms such as spots, flashes (photopsia), flickering (scintillations) and zig-zags (teichopsia) or negative symptoms including patchy or homonymous loss of vision (scotomota and heminanopia).
- Typical sensory aura is unilateral and also may be positive (tingling) or negative (numbness) and should be differentiated from true motor weakness
- Speech disturbance is characterized by non-fluent dysphasia.
- Typical aura should not last longer than 60min.
- Migraine headache usual starts within 1h of aura onset or resolution

Aura without headache

- Aura symptoms in the absence of headache occur in 20–44% of migraine sufferers.
- Population prevalence is ~1%. 77% begin after age 50 years and 40% have no prior history of headache.
- Visual aura symptoms are the most common clinical symptom. More frequent between 40 and 60 years of age and have been termed 'late life migraine accompaniments'. Individuals usually have a prior history of migraine, usually MA.
- Aura without headache can occur in isolation and, if associated with vascular risk factors, later life onset and especially if starting abruptly, must be differentiated from a TIA.

Hemiplegic migraine

- Migraine aura sometimes includes motor weakness that may involve facial paresis, monoparesis (most commonly the upper limb) and hemiparesis.
- Less commonly motor aura may consist of simultaneous bilateral limb weakness.
- Hemiplegic migraine has both familial (FHM) and sporadic forms (SHM). The diagnostic criteria for each variant form of hemiplegic migraine are shown in Table 4.9.
- The diagnosis is only tenable when there is no other diagnosis that would explain these symptoms.
- Both forms are indistinguishable clinically and can only be distinguished diagnostically by the absence of a first- or second-degree relative with motor aura.
- In SHM there is thus sometimes the need to not only exclude secondary mimics for SHM but also to examine the proband's extended family to identify similar sufferers

Clinical features of FHM and SHM

- The prevalence of hemiplegic migraine is ~0.001%.
- SHM and FHM are thought to have equal prevalence and more commonly affect the female sex.
- Hemiplegic migraine occurs first usually in childhood or mid to late adolescence (mean 12–17 years of age). 97% occur by age 45 years
- Hemiplegic attacks 'stop' in later life but may continue as conventional attacks of migraine with or without aura or aura without headache.
- It is very unusual for motor aura to occur in isolation without other aura symptoms. Other forms of aura occur in order of relative frequency: sensory aura > visual aura > dysphasia.
- Up to 20% of attacks are associated with symptoms and signs of impaired consciousness, and sometimes encephalopathy or coma.
- In up to 60% aura may last longer than 60 min, and 8% have attacks which last days before recovery.
- Sufferers also experience intervening attacks of more common migraine with or without aura attacks. MA attacks may have more prolonged aura symptoms. Attacks of basilar type migraine aura occur in 2/3 of individuals.

Table 4.9 Familial and sporadic hemiplegic migraine ICHD-II diagnostic criteria

Familial hemiplegic migraine can be diagnosed clinically when individuals experience ≥2 attacks of:

- Aura consisting of fully reversible motor weakness and at least 1 symptom of:
  - Fully reversible visual aura symptoms and/or
  - Fully reversible sensory aura symptoms and/or
  - Fully reversible aura symptoms of dysphasia
- Where at least one of the following:
  - Aura symptoms either develop gradually over ≥5min and/or different aura symptoms occur in rapid succession over ≥5min
  - Each aura symptom lasts ≥5 min and <24h
  - The above features are associated with characteristic migraine headache during the aura or within 1h of aura onset
- At least 1 other 1st or 2nd degree relative has attacks fulfilling the criteria above

Sporadic hemiplegic migraine can be diagnosed when the above criteria are fulfilled and there are no family members with similar attacks

Table 4.10 Differential diagnosis of hemiplegic migraine

- Cerebrovascular disease
  - TIAs and ischaemic stroke
  - AVMs and intracerebral haemorrhage
  - Cervical and cerebral arterial dissection
  - Coagulopathies (e.g. antiphospholipid syndrome)
  - Cerebral vasculitis
- Epileptic seizures with Todd's paresis
- Meningoencephalitis
- Rare inherited disorders
  - Mitochondrial disease (MELAS)
  - CADASIL (cerebral autosomal dominant arteriopathy with subcortical infarcts and leukoencephalopathy)
- HaNDL (syndrome of transient headache and neurological deficits with CSF lymphocytosis)
- Metabolic disorders
  - Severe electrolyte disturbance
  - Homocystinuria
- Ornithine transcarbamylase deficiency

Genetics of familial hemiplegic migraine

- FHM is inherited as an autosomal-dominant genetic disorder and is the only migraine variant to have pathogenic gene mutations identified.
- The 3 genes identified are all involved in modulating ion channel function (see Table 4.11).
- FHM mutations lower the threshold required to produce cortical spreading depression and increase cortical excitability.
- Genetic screening of SHM sufferers does not identify FHM genotypes despite their clinical similarities, and has no place in conventional clinic management at present.
- Subgroups of FHM1 may develop a progressive cerebellar ataxic syndrome (SCA-6).
- A rare FHM phenotype due a point mutation in the CACNA1A gene (serine-218-leucine) is associated with FHM and associated fatal coma in the context of minor head trauma triggering fatal cerebral oedema.

Treatment of familial hemiplegic migraine

- There are no RCTs of therapy in hemiplegic migraine.
- As individuals also experience attacks of migraine with and without aura, conventional migraine prophylaxis is appropriate.
- Triptans are relatively contraindicated in hemiplegic migraine since there is insufficient systematic evidence. Expert advice is appropriate.
- Some authors advocate the following unlicensed agents in addition to the usual first-line migraine preventative agents.
  - Verapamil 120–360mg daily
  - Acetazolamide 500mg daily
  - Flunarizine 5–10mg

Basilar-type migraine

- Attacks where aura symptoms imply reversible brainstem dysfunction.
- Aura is thought to originate from brainstem structures and/or bilateral simultaneous cerebral hemisphere involvement in the absence of motor weakness.
- Occurs in up to 10% of MA sufferers and may occur in any sufferer of MA. More than 90% of patients who suffer basilar-type migraine also have attacks of more typical MA.
- Basilar-type migraine aura symptoms are more common in patients with either FHM or SHM as part of their hemiplegic attacks. Thus the presence of motor weakness during aura in such individuals implies a diagnosis of hemiplegic migraine.
- The presence of a family history or a history of recurrent attacks of MA or prior migraine with reversible hemiparesis obviates the need for extensive investigation.
- Treatment is as for hemiplegic migraine.

Table 4.11 Summary of FHM genetic subtypes

Familial hemiplegic subtype	FHM 1	FHM 2	FHM 3
Chromosome	19p13	1q23	2q24
Gene involved	CACNA1A	ATP1A2	SCN1A
Ion channel subunit encoded	α-1 subnit Ca$_v$1.2 (P/Q)	A1A2 Na$^+$/ K$^+$ATPase	α-1 subnit Na$_v$1.1
% of FHM families involved (approx)	50–70%	20–30%	Unknown
Inter attacks of cerebellar signs*	50%	Some (frequency?)	None

* Cerebellar signs characterized by persisting nystagmus, gait and/or limb ataxia, dysarthria.

Table 4.12 Basilar-type migraine ICHD-II diagnostic criteria

Two or more attacks of:
- At least 2 fully reversible aura symptoms manifest as:
  - Dysarthria
  - Diplopia
  - Vertigo
  - Tinnitus
  - Hyperaccusis
  - Ataxia
  - Reduced level of consciousness
  - Simultaneous whole visual field aura symptoms
  - Bilateral simultaneous sensory aura symptoms
- No focal motor weakness
- Aura should be characterized by at least one of the following:
  - Aura symptoms either develop gradually over ≥5min and/or different aura symptoms occur in rapid succession over ≥5min
  - Each aura symptom lasts ≥5min and <24h
  - The above features are associated with characteristic migraine headache during the aura or within 1h of aura onset

Retinal migraine
- Previously know as 'ocular migraine'.
- Characterized by monocular visual symptomotology in contrast to usual binocular visual aura symptoms in MA.
- Visual symptoms include monocular:
  - Scotomota
  - Heminanopia
  - Photopsia
  - Pupillary abnormalities
- Exclude monocular visual disturbance due to retro-orbital lesion, TIAs temporal arteritis.

Childhood periodic syndromes
These variants affect children and adolescents in early life. They describe recurrent episodic symptoms (usually in the absence of headache) that are associated with the development of migraine in adult life (see Table 4.13)

Other variants of migraine (not currently in the IHS classification)
Although not included in the ICHD-II migraine classification, several clinical syndromes are described as potentially within the spectrum of migraine

Vestibular migraine/migrainous vertigo (MV)
- Also known as migrainous vertigo, migraine-related vertigo, migraine-associated dizziness, but no uniform nomenclature adopted.
- Diagnosis is clinical and should be differentiated from other causes of episodic vertigo, e.g. vertigo as an aura symptom occurring in the context of a basilar-type migraine variant.
- Population prevalence of migrainous vertigo may be 1% and symptoms begin at any age.
- Clinical characteristics and differential diagnosis are shown in Table 4.14 and 4.15.
- Treatment
  - Short-term use of symptomatic medication for acute symptoms of vertigo and nausea (neuroleptics and antiemetics).

Prophylactic migraine medications are unproven but advocated on anecdotal response rates. β-Blockers, TCAs and calcium channel blockers have all been used.

Table 4.13 Childhood periodic syndromes

Cyclic vomiting

- Usually a family history of migraine.
- Symptoms often begin in the middle of the night. Girls more affected than boys.
- Begins at ~5 years of age; resolves in 50% by 10 years and most by puberty.
- Recurrent stereotyped attacks (>5) of severe nausea and vomiting associated with pallor, lethargy ± autonomic symptoms.
- Explosive, frequent attacks of nausea and vomiting lasting hours to days
- Symptom free between attacks.
- History and examination do not show signs of gastrointestinal disease, intermittent bowel obstruction and metabolic disorders, e.g. hereditary aminoacidurias, organic acidaemias, fatty acid oxidation disorders and porphyria.
- Treated with antiemetics, rehydration. Conventional migraine preventative effective in reducing attacks frequency.

Abdominal migraine

- Also known as cyclic abdominal pain but is less common and less severe than cyclic vomiting.
- More common in children aged 7–13 years with a family history of migraine.
- Recurrent, episodic, attacks (>5) lasting 1h up to 3 days.
- Abdominal pain has a dull character usually in a midline periumbilical location but can be more diffuse. Pain is sufficiently severe to affect daily activities.
- At least 2 symptoms of anorexia, nausea, vomiting or pallor are present.
- Treatment is with conventional migraine preventative medication.

Benign paroxysmal vertigo of childhood

- More commonly affects young children. Attacks begin suddenly, last minutes only and may occur in clusters lasting days to weeks.
- Paroxysmal, recurrent, untriggered, attacks of severe vertigo ± gait unsteadiness without warning.
- During attacks the child may:
- Appear frightened and find difficulty maintaining balance
- Have nystagmus during the attack but normal neurological examination between attacks
- Have associated pallor, nausea ± vomiting
- Vestibular function tests between attacks are normal, excluding peripheral vestibular disease.
- If no atypical features and rapid symptom resolution, then no investigations are needed. If persistent or additional brainstem symptoms or atypical or persistent signs, then brain MRI to exclude secondary pathology.
- The relationship between benign paroxysmal vertigo and later life so-called vestibular migraine that occurs in adulthood is not yet clear.

Benign paroxysmal torticollis (of infancy)

An uncommon disorder of infancy and early childhood. It begins in the first year of life and may evolve into benign paroxysmal vertigo of childhood or migraine with aura. Can cease altogether before 5 years of age.

- Recurrent episodes of head tilt (torticollis) ± head rotation
- Torticollis may alternate sides
- Torticollis last minutes to days and infant/child well between attacks
- May be associated pallor, irritability, nausea and vomiting
- The differential diagnosis includes infantile dystonia, complex partial seizures and congenital lesions of the foramen magnum.
- Brain MRI, EEG and, if appropriate, dystonia screening may be needed.

'Alice in Wonderland syndrome'

Clinical syndrome of complex visual phenomena as part of visual aura. Most often seen in children and may occur in the absence of headache

- Bizarre visual hallucinations and visual distortions usually precede migraine headache.
- Hallucinations, illusions include macropsia, micropsia (*objects appear larger or smaller than they actually are*), spatial distortions such as metamorphopsia or teleopsia (*visual error in judging distances of objects in space*).
- There is no accompanying confusion, and awareness is preserved during visual symptoms.
- Exclude psychotropic drug intoxication and occipital epilepsy.

Confusional migraine

Characterized by disorientation, confusion, sometimes with agitation, restlessness and impaired awareness in the setting of an attack of migraine with or without aura.

- Attacks more common in adolescents than adults,
- May be precipitated by mild head trauma and more often occur in the context of a hemiplegic or basilar-type migraine attack,
- Recovery usually occurs within 4–6h and should be associated with typical migraine headache and associated symptomatology,
- Investigations are warranted for a first attack especially if no prior history of migraine.
- Brain MRI imaging is usually normal, but EEG changes, i.e slow wave activity, may be seen during the attack.
- Drug intoxication, complex partial epilepsy and metabolic encephalopathy may need to be excluded.

Treatment consists of conventional migraine prophylaxis if attacks are recurrent.

Menstrual migraine

- See Chapter 6.

Table 4.14 Clinical characteristics of vestibular migraine

- Episodic features include
  - Spontaneous illusion of movement, i.e vertigo
  - Rotational or 'to-and-fro' sensations
  - Positional vertigo
  - Visual vertigo (provoked by busy moving scenes)
  - Postural imbalance
- Vertiginous symptoms highly variable in duration and frequency
  - Seconds to weeks duration
  - More common minutes to hours
  - Monthly or yearly frequency or clusters over a few days
- Associated symptoms
  - May occur variably with/without headache
  - 50% never have an associated headache—vertigo only manifestation of migraine
  - MA is the predominant migraine subtype at other times when vertigo is not present
  - Photophobia, phonophobia, osmophobia are commonly present if questioned

Table 4.15 Differential diagnosis of vestibular migraine

- BPPV—positional triggered vertigo and positive Dix–Hallpike test
- Menieres disease—sensorineural deafness, aural fullness & tinnitus
- Central positional vertigo, e.g. multiple sclerosis, stroke—other brainstem symptoms and signs
- Vestibular paroxysmia—brief, recurrent, seconds duration only
- Panic disorder—autonomic, anxiety and avoidance behaviour, and scenario specific

Migraine as part of a neurological syndrome

Both CADASIL and MELAS can sometimes be mistakenly diagnosed as hemiplegic migraine so a high index of suspicion is needed if the relevant associated clinical features are identified (see Table 4.16).

Complications of migraine

Chronic migraine

- Headache is on 15 days or more per month for >3 months in the absence of analgesic medication overuse.
- Affects ~2% of migraine sufferers and has a significant impact on the quality of life.
- Has the clinical characteristics of migraine (usually without aura) on at least 8 of these days per month or responds to a triptan or ergot if used early during the headache phase.
- No other cause of frequent headache is identifiable.
- Diagnosis of chronic migraine can only be established when the required pattern continues after analgesic overuse cessation for >4–8 weeks.

Status migrainous

- A migraine attack that lasts longer than 3 days is described as 'status migrainous'.
- An attack lasting >7 days may be a better time point to define status migrainosis as alerts to the need for clinical review to exclude secondary headache.
- History of headache onset should be reviewed and caution should be exercised particularly additional and/or persistent neurological symptoms or signs, e.g. cervical extracranial arterial dissection causing persistent unilateral migraine like headache with anterior neck pain and ipsilateral Horner's syndrome.
- Usually occurs as part of the spectrum of migraine, but exact pathogenic mechanism not clear.
- May reflect central thalamic activation of migraine pain pathways (central sensitization).
- Extended use of acute ergot, triptan or other analgesics to treat the acute attack may be an alternative reason.

Migrainous infarction

- True migrainous infarction is extremely rare, and the true frequency is unknown.
- Probably overdiagnosed. A recent study suggests 0.5–1% of all strokes are due to migrainous infarction.
- Migrainous infarction most frequently occurs in the posterior cerebral artery territory (as aura is most commonly visual).
- The exact pathogenic mechanism is unclear.

Table 4.16 Migraine as part of a neurological syndrome

Cerebral autosomal dominant arteriopathy with subcortical infarcts and leukoencephalopathy (CADASIL)

Rare autosomal dominant neurological disorder due to mutations in the NOTCH 3 gene on chromosome 19p13. The gene mutation is associated with eosinophilic deposits in vascular smooth muscle and skin, and is characterized by a microangiopathy affecting the brain.

- 90% have migraine with aura. Onset in the mid-20s is often the first manifestation.
- Stroke-like episodes in 85% of sufferers before age 60
  - Present as lacunar TIAs an stroke syndromes
  - Mean age at stroke onset mid-40s
- Cognitive deficits and dementia in 60% at onset
  - Dementia affects 75% of sufferers
  - Executive function, language and memory most affected
- Psychiatric disorder including pesonality change and depression
- Brain MRI abnormalities consistently seen after age 21
  - Temporal lobe high T2 white matter lesions
  - External capsule high T2 white matter lesions
  - Subcortical lacunar lesions and cerebral microbleeds
- Epilepsy in 10% of sufferers presents by middle age

Mitochondrial encephalamyopathy, lactic acidosis and stroke-like episodes (MELAS)

A multisystem disorder caused by a gene mutation in mitochondrial DNA (mtDNA).

- Usually due to maternal transmission and onset of symptoms usually begin in adolescence or childhood.
- Stroke-like episodes before age 40 years
- Encephalopathy with seizures ± dementia
- Mitochondrial myopathy
- Recurrent migraine-like headache
- Lactic acidosis (increased lactate and pyruvate levels)
- Brain MRI abnormalities during acute stroke-like episodes
  - Non-vascular territory posterior cerebral high T2 signal lesions
  - Basal ganglia calcification on brain CT

Other clinical features include:

- Short stature
- Epilepsy (tonic–clonic and myoclonic seizures)
- Sensorineural deafness
- Diabetes mellitus
- Cardiomyopathy
- Neuropathy
- Ataxia
- Dementia
- Progressive external ophthalmoplegia or optic neuropathy
- Gastrointestinal dysfunction/dysmotility

Minimum investigations to be performed before making a diagnosis of migrainous infarction should include:

- Brain MRI ± intracranial and carotid/vertebral MRA (or CT angiography)
- Antiphospholipid syndrome studies
- Prothombotic coagulation studies
- Transoesophogeal echocardiography
- Consideration of gene studies for CADASIL and MELAS

IHS criteria for migrainous infarction are:

- The individual has a prior established history of migraine with aura
- The cerebral infarct occurs during an attack of typical migraine with aura
- A clinically relevant area of brain infarction is identified on brain imaging
- There is no other alternative cause for the stroke (headache may occur in the context of typical ischaemic stroke)

Persistent aura without infarction

- Aura symptoms typically last <1hour in up to 95% of the population who experience MA.
- Less commonly attacks of aura (and especially sensory or paretic aura) are more prolonged.
- Persistent aura should prompt early investigation unless there is an established stereotyped pattern or there is a family history of similar episodes to suggest FHM.
- Secondary disorders that can manifest as unusual aura include:
  - Occipital or cortical AVMs
  - Vertex meningiomas situated on the somatosensory or motor cortex
  - Syndromes where atypically prolonged aura is a more common event, e.g. CADASIL

Migraine-triggered seizures

- Sometimes termed 'migralepsy' this describes the scenario of a seizure occurring during or immediately following a migraine attack.
- It reportedly affects ~2–3% of individuals diagnosed with both migraine and epilepsy.

Migraine aura status

- Aura usually occurs as a monophasic event and most commonly precedes or occurs during the migraine headache phase.
- Aura can occur in the absence of headache.
- Rarely migraine aura (usually visual) can occur on multiple occasions per day and even on consecutive days during an attack.
- Recently suggested criteria are typical migraine aura occurring up to twice per day for ≥5 consecutive days
- Secondary headache disorders should be excluded.

When to investigate

The amount of investigation beyond a good history and neurological examination in migraine should be proportionate to the nature (typical or atypical), frequency and duration of attacks. In general terms with a firm diagnosis of migraine and a normal examination there is no indication to investigate.

Consider more extensive investigations when:
- Patients present for the first time with a rare migraine subtype especially when there is no prior established history of such attacks.
  - Hemiplegic migraine
  - Basilar-type migraine
  - Retinal migraine
  - Migraine aura status
  - Vestibular migraine
- Patients present with aura symptoms that do not resolve within 24h, i.e prolonged aura suggesting stroke or focal brain insult or where there is impaired consciousness with the attack
- A dramatic change or unexplained increase in migraine aura symptoms
- An abrupt onset to aura with (ipsilateral) headache and a Horner's syndrome (cervical arterial dissection?)
- Associated strong autosomal dominant family history of young onset stroke (<50 years), Dementia in middle age (40–60 years), Depression and migraine with prolonged aura or hemiplegia (CADASIL)
- Associated multisystem disease. e.g. sensorineural deafness, short stature, ataxia, ophthalmoplegia, myopathy, diabetes and stroke-like events with migraine with aura.

How to investigate

- The investigation of migraine is determined by the history, examination and what is considered to be the most likely alternative 'migraine variant mimic'.
- An awareness of the false-positive and false-negative limitations of routine blood testing is essential.
- Match relevant MRI and interpretation to clinical symptoms. Be clear about your concerns on the request form.
- The following investigations are sometimes useful in the evaluation of migraine and its variants, but it is essential to be guided by the clinical syndrome and suspected alternative diagnosis rather than simply perform investigations as part of a 'fishing trip'!

Common
- Full blood count and platelets
- APPT, INR (± coagulation profile) and ESR
- Biochemical profile and glucose
- ANF, dsDNA, anticardiolipin antibodies and lupus anticoagulant
- Brain MRI and MRA (cerebral and neck vessels) MRV
- Lumbar puncture.

Rarer
- Toxicology screen
- EEG
- Plasma (± CSF lactate)
- Carotid Doppler
- Cardiac echo
- Mitochondrial DNA, NOTCH 3 genotyping (± skin biopsy).

Migraine treatment

Behaviour and lifestyle modification

The migraine attack is triggered by the complex interplay of many factors. Identification can offer treatment and management strategies. Triggers can be direct chemical or environmental change. Migraineurs find it difficult to react to changes in environmental inputs, both internal and external.

Migraine triggers

- The mode of action of most triggers is poorly understood.
- The role of allergy remains contested.
- Apart from direct action, triggers may alter migraine threshold.
- Triggers interact with each other and environment factors, and therefore action is not consistent.
- As migraine and trigger exposure may be frequent, a causal relationship may be incorrectly deduced.
- Premonitory symptoms of migraine, e.g. chocolate craving, may be mistaken for a trigger.
- Important triggers may be constituents of drugs taken for headache or foodstuffs. The latter is particularly important in children (see Tables 5.1 and 5.2).
- Triggers should be avoided only when a reliable pattern is established.

Environmental factors

Keeping the headache threshold high

A full understanding of patients' lifestyle is needed. The right questions result in the right support and empower the patient to consider and implement relevant change.

Areas to explore are:

- Occupation
  - Shift patterns
  - Overtime
  - Ergonomics of workplace
  - Use of telephones, computers, etc.
  - Hours spent driving
  - Regular meal breaks
  - Time and target management issues
  - Interpersonal conflicts
- Family
  - Health and family illness
  - Being a carer
  - Child care
  - Relationship issues

Table 5.1 Caffeine content of painkillers that can be purchased in the UK without prescription

Name of preparation	Caffeine content
Alka-Seltzer XS®	40mg
Anadin Extra®	45mg
Boots Tension Headache Relief®	30mg
Hedex Extra®	65mg
Panadol Extra®	65mg
Phensic Original®	22mg
Propain®	50mg
Solpadeine Plus®	30mg
Syndol®	30mg

Table 5.2 Caffeine content of drinks and chocolate

Item	Item size	Caffeine content
Coffee	150ml (5oz)	60–150mg
Coffee, decaffeinated	150ml (5oz)	2–5mg
Tea	150ml (5oz)	40–80mg
Cocoa	150ml (5oz)	1–8mg
Coca Cola®	12oz	64mg
Diet Coca Cola®	12oz	45mg
Dr Pepper®	12oz	61mg
Pepsi Cola®	12oz	43mg
Kit-Kat® bar	1 bar, 47g	5mg
Chocolate brownie	1.25oz	8mg
Chocolate ice cream	50g	2–5mg
Milk chocolate	1oz	1.15mg
Special dark chocolate bar	1 bar, 41g	31mg
After Eight® mint	2 pieces, 8g	1.6mg

- Lifestyle
  - Exercise
  - Healthy diet
  - Regular meals and healthy snacks
  - Caffeine intake
  - Water intake
  - Alcohol and recreational drugs
  - Stress at home and work
  - 'Me' time and hobbies

Understanding and facilitating the process of change

Figure 5.1 shows an approach to change management. Change is unlikely to occur unless there is an understanding of the influences that affect change and the intervention is matched to the stage of the patient within a context of a supportive environment.

- The context of change
  - Social and cultural features: expectations based on personal and family relationships, age, gender, social class, ethnicity, ability to access information and knowledge which will affect ability to contemplate or initiate change. Change that fits within the cultural norm will be more readily accepted.
  - Ethical and spiritual features: personal and shared values and moral systems from which these values are derived. Include rituals, religion and rights of passage.
  - Political and legal features: determine what can and can't be done and define limits to social change.
  - Resource features: what resources are needed to make change happen. This may cover human, financial as well as practical or physical resources essential to enable change to occur.
  - Personality: understanding the personality type in front of you will help you and the patient make the effective choices and decisions. People will adopt change depending upon where they are in absorbing and processing an idea or concept.

Some concepts to help change happen

- Change is more likely to happen if there is a 'relative advantage' of the new behavior (drinking more water) over existing behavior (drinking lots of fresh coffee). The new behavior has to feel compatible with their normal day-to-day activities, within their home, social or work environment.
- The less complex the change, the more likely it is to be adopted especially if it can be used for a trial period to assess its effectiveness.
- Small changes may have the greatest impact - make change doable and achievable.
- Set priorities for change—identify relevant goals.
- Support the change.

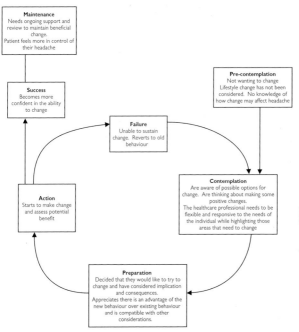

Fig. 5.1 The process of change (after Prochaska and DiClemente). Match the intervention to the stages of change. A patient may go through a number of cycles before change is maintained. Adapted from Prochaska J, DiClemente C. (1998). Towards a comprehensive model of change. In: Miller WR, Heather N (Eds). *Treating addictive behaviours: processes of change.* New York: Plenum.

Practical tips to reduce migraine

- Start the day with a cereal, ideally oat based. A low glycaemic index cereal offers a slow release of sugar to keep the headache patient going until lunchtime.
- Eat three meals a day, or even more frequently with smaller portions. Do not go longer than 4h in the daytime and 12h overnight without something to eat.
- Avoid known trigger foods and drinks
- Limit your caffeine consumption, well below 200mg a day. Watch both food and analgesia for caffeine.
- Avoid eating excessive amounts of carbohydrates, fats, protein or sugars at any one sitting. Caution with junk foods, processed sugars, sweets and biscuits.
- Ensure an adequate fluid intake, ideally 2 litres of water each day.
- All things in moderation, even alcohol.
- Avoid prolonged stress or anxiety: the 'let down' after stress can trigger a headache; regular breaks in the day reduce the build up of stress; plan in some 'me' time.
- Encourage a consistent sleep pattern. Too much or too little sleep can trigger headache. Have a bedtime snack or keep a snack by the bed for when first waking. If working shifts, try and eat and drink regularly to reduce the effect of a changing sleep pattern.
- Avoid multiple triggers.
- Watch out for poor posture
  - Ergonomics: home or work
  - If using a phone, is there a headset?
  - Reduce exposure to computer games, monitor use of laptops.
  - Think about driving position
- Understand and modify drug-taking behaviour
  - Poor previous experience
  - Lack of understanding of drug action
  - Reluctance to take regular medication
  - Stigma attached to drugs, e.g. TCAs and depression

Table 5.3 Ten key tips for patient to raise their headache threshold

- Eat regular meals
- Avoid known trigger foods and drinks
- Avoid prolonged fasting, avoid hunger
- Ensure adequate fluid intake, avoid thirst
- Be consistent in your sleep habits
- Avoid stress where possible
- Treat your attack as early as possible
- Take your medication as prescribed
- Avoid multiple triggers
- Don't be afraid to ask for advice and help

Pharmacological treatment of the acute attack

With the exception of the triptans, the evidence base for acute treatment is limited. Appendix 5 provides some important drug interactions.

Stepped or stratified treatment?

Three acute treatment options exist.
- Stepped care within the attack, i.e. starting with simple analgesics. If ineffective, moving towards stronger drugs.
- Stepped care between attacks. This is the same approach but increasing medication with consecutive attacks.
- Stratified care, matching the approach to the severity of the attack.

A pragmatic option is to explain to the patient treatment options and allow them to establish what is best for them.

Simple analgesia/anti-inflammatory/prokinetic agent

- A useful first step is paracetamol 1000mg, ibuprofen 400–600mg and domperidone 10mg. These can be bought without prescription.
  - If the patient is unsure whether the headache will develop into a migraine, this is a useful option prior to taking a triptan.
  - Higher doses taken initially will facilitate a more rapid attainment of therapeutic levels. Maximum recommended doses should not be exceeded over a 24h period.
  - Soluble or dispersible preparations have theoretically quicker uptake.
  - Even if nausea is not present, domperidone will help to negate the impact of gastric stasis on absorption.
  - Metoclopramide (10mg) is an alternative to domperidone but side effects particularly dyskinaesia can be more severe and a prescription is needed.
  - Metoclopramide combination products are more convenient but more expensive (MigraMax® with asprin (900/10mg) and Paramax® with paracetamol (500/5mg)).

Rectal NSAID/prokinetic agent

If severe nausea or vomiting, diclofenac 100mg suppositories (up to 200mg in 24h) and domperidone 30mg suppositories (up to 120mg in 24h) can be used. This can be repeated after 4h.

Ergots

- Ergots have historically been the mainstay of migraine treatment, but have been superseded by triptans.
- Act as 5-HT agonists but wide range of other actions limit use.
- Significant side effects include nausea, dizziness, paraesthesia, abdominal pain, chest tightness

Table 5.4 The emergency migraine call out

- The first attack can cause diagnostic concern and often leads to an admission to exclude meningitis or SAH.
- Subcutaneous sumatriptan is the treatment of choice, but is rarely carried in a GP bag.
- Avoid opiates—patients rapidly become dependent on them
- Use IM diclofenac (50mg) combined with an antiemetic (prochlorperazine 12.5mg or metoclopramide 10mg).
- Sort out the migraine. A subsequent emergency call out reflects a failure of adequate management.

Table 5.5 Criteria for admission

- The first attack of migraine where there is diagnostic uncertainty. (particularly relevant for certain migraine variants such as hemiplegic migraine, migrainous infarction, basilar-type migraine.
- When there is a suspicion of an underlying vascular episode (stroke, aneurysm, SAH, carotid dissection).
- Headache associated with intractable vomiting producing dehydration.

Table 5.6 Status migrainosis

- IV fluids
- IV prochlorperazine 10mg or metoclopramide 10mg
- IV dihydroergotamine 0.5–1mg IV. Repeat 0.5mg after 1h if BP stable
- Consider dexamethasone 4mg, IV diazepam 5–10mg

- Rectal absorption is more predictable than oral
- Contraindications of pregnancy, uncontrolled hypertension, renal or hepatic failure and arterial disease.
- Rebound can be a problem.
- Useful if patients are intolerant to triptans.

Ergotamine preparations include:
- Oral ergotamine 1–2mg (unpredictable absorption). Max 4 tabs in any attack, no more than twice a month. Available as Cafergot® (ergotamine 1mg/100mg caffeine) and Migril® (ergotamine 2mg/ cyclizine 50mg/caffeine 100mg.)
- Ergotamine suppository. Better absorption. Available as Cafergot® suppositories (ergotamine 2mg/caffeine 100mg). Max 2 in 24h
- Dihydroergotamine nasal spray 2mg.
- Dihydroergotamine IM/SC 1mg.

Triptans

Triptans were designed to mimic the effect of serotonin without its side effects and act on $5HT_1$ receptors across the trigeminovascular system. There is a large evidence base underpinning their use, and much effort is spent in attempts to differentiate them for marketing purposes.
- Patients will vary in their response to triptans. 30% of patients will fail to respond. There is a >70% chance that an alternative triptan will be successful. The basis for this observation is not understood.
- Can be taken with analgesia/NSAID/prokinetic drugs but not ergots.
- Triptans should not be taken too early in the attack. There is a suggestion that they do not work effectively if taken during the aura phase.
- A second dose can be taken after 2h providing there has been a response to the first dose. Maximum 2 doses in 24h. (These are licensing requirements rather than practical or theoretical concerns.)
- All triptans are associated with a recurrence in 30% of patients (return of symptoms within 48h following initial response).
- A rebound headache (related to the mode of triptan action and not the migraine progression) can occur in up to 30% of patients.
- A synergistic effect has been demonstrated with naproxen 500mg.

Table 5.7 A comparison of the action of ergotamine and sumatriptan on receptor affinity. Different triptans will have a different spectrum of activity across 5-HT1 sites. The wider action of ergotamine accounts for its greater incidence of side effects

Site	Agonists	
	Ergotamine	Sumatriptan
5-HT		+
1A	+++	++
1B	++	++
1D	++	−
1E	++	++
1F	+	−
2	+	−
3	−	−
Adrenergic		
α1	+	−
α2	+	−
β	±	−
Dopaminergic	±	

Table 5.8 Triptan delivery modes

Preparation	Drug	Indication
Parenteral	Sumatriptan 6mg SC	Severe vomiting, rapidly developing symptoms
Nasal	Sumatriptan 10mg and 20mg nasal spray, zolmitriptan nasal spray 5mg	Useful where vomiting or severe nausea is a problem. Approximately 20% gets absorbed through the nose
Oral	All triptans. Melts and wafers are for convenience only and do not get absorbed through the oral mucosa. Dispersible preparations offer theoretically increased rate of absorption	

- Unlicensed for >65 years. This is due to the concern of an increased possibility of underlying vascular disease. However, in some cases the benefits may outweigh the potential risks. A prior ECG is recommended.
- The origin of the chest pain seen with triptans remains unclear. It may be oesophageal or pulmonary artery spasm.

Contraindications

Ischaemic heart disease, previous myocardial infarction, coronary vasospasm, uncontrolled or severe hypertension, cerebral vascular disease, peripheral vascular disease, breastfeeding, pregnancy.

Side effects

Sensations of tingling, heat, heaviness, pressure, chest pain, flushing, dizziness, weakness, fatigue, nausea and vomiting.

Drug interactions

- Clarithromycin and erythromycin raise plasma concentrations of eletriptan.
- Quinolones raise plasma concentration of zolmitriptan.
- Increased serotonergic effect with St John's Wort.
- Plasma concentration of eletriptan and almotriptan increased by oral antifungals.
- Plasma concentration of rizatriptan increased by propranolol (use half dose of rizatriptan).
- Avoid ergot alkaloids—increases the risk of vasospasm (ergotamine and methysergide).
- Cimetidine increases plasma concentration of zolmitriptan.
- SSRIs. Theoretical risk of serotonin syndrome.
  - Serotonin syndrome ranges from gastrointestinal complaints, tremor, muscle rigidity, cognitive change to very rarely death.
  - In the USA, 20% of migraineurs are taking an SSRI with a triptan
  - The annual incidence of serotonin syndrome with co-exposure is <0.03%. This is less than the incidence with SSRIs alone.
  - The combination of SSRI/triptan is not contraindicated but must be given with caution.

Opiates

Due to side effects and potential for addiction, only use in specialized circumstances. Rebound headache is a problem. Can be used for severe headaches that are relatively infrequent where other agents have failed. Useful in intractable menstrual migraine or during pregnancy.

Steroids

Can be useful to abort chronic migraine or migraine that has become out of control.

- 1mg/kg of prednisolone up to a maximum of 60mg for 1 week, reducing over 4 weeks.
- Maximum number of courses three times a year.
- Main side effects over this time period are CNS disturbances:
  - Hypomania
  - Psychosis
  - Depression.

Table 5.9 Some considerations when using triptans (based on). Comparison is with 100mg sumatriptan

	Initial 2h relief	Sustained pain free	Consistency	Tolerability
Sumatriptan 50mg	=	=	=/–	=
Sumatriptan 25mg	–	=/–	–	+
Zolmitriptan 2.5mg	=	=	=	=
Zolmitriptan 5mg	=	=	=	=
Naratriptan 2.5mg	–	–	–	++
Rizatriptan 5mg	=	=	=	=
Rizatriptan 10mg	+	+	++	=
Eletriptan 20mg	–	–	–	=
Eletriptan 40mg	=/+	=/+	=	=
Eletriptan 80mg	+	+	=	–
Almotriptan 12.5mg	=	+	+	++
Frovatriptan 2.5mg	–	=	=	++

Ferari MD, et al. (2001). Oral triptans (serotonin 5HR (1B/1D) agonists) in acute migraine treatment: a meta-analysis of 53 trials. *Lancet.* **358**: 1668-75.

Table 5.10 A pragmatic approach to choosing a triptan (choose the cheapest drug in each group)

Triptans with a shorter half-life (quicker initial relief)	Triptans with a longer half-life (lower side effect profile and theoretically less recurrence)
Sumatriptan	Frovatriptan
Zolmitriptan	Eletriptan
Naratriptan	
Rizatriptan	
Almotriptan	

- Other concerns are
  - Unmasking of underlying diabetes
  - Insomnia
  - Immune suppression in susceptible patients
  - Use with caution if systemic infection present.

Nausea and vomiting

This can be more disabling than headache. Triggering of central mechanisms and gastrointestinal stasis are the predominant mechanisms. Figure 5.2 shows mechanisms of nausea and vomiting, and Table 5.11 shows receptor site affinities of antiemetics.

- Domperidone (10mg oral, 30 mg suppository)
- Metoclopramide (10mg oral and 10mg IM) act predominately on gastric stasis.
- Promethazine, chlorpromazine, prochlorperazine (5mg oral, 3mg buccal, 25 mg suppository, 12.5mg IM) act predominately centrally.
- Ondansetron (8mg oral) can be used where vomiting is severe, and acts centrally and peripherally.

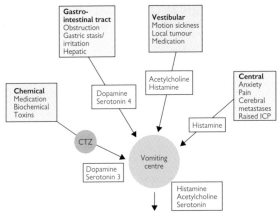

Fig. 5.2 Mechanisms of nausea and vomiting and suggested receptors and neurotransmitters involved. Reproduced with permission from Watson et al. (2005). *Oxford Handbook of Palliative Care.* Oxford University Press.

Table 5.11 Receptor site affinities of antiemetics

	D$_2$ antagonist	H$_1$ antagonist	Ach antagonist	5-HT$_3$ antagonist
Metoclopramide	++	0	0	(+)
Ondansetron	0	0	0	+++
Cyclzine	0	++	++	0
Hyoscine hydrobromide	0	0	+++	0
Haloperidol	+++	0	0	0
Prochlorperazine	++	+	0	0
Chlorpromazine	++	++	+	0
Levomepromazine	++	+++	++	0

D$_1$ =doparmine, H$_2$ = histamine1, Ach =muscannic cholinergic, 5-HT$_3$ = serotonin group 3

* Adapted from Twycross R, Back I, Nausea and vomiting in advanced cancer. *European J of Pali Care* 1998, 5: 39–45.

Pharmacological treatment for prevention

Preventive medications are used to reduce the frequency, duration or severity of migraine attacks. There are no rules as to when they should be started, but factors that should be taken into account in conjunction with the patient are:

- If there is significant headache-related disability.
- When too much acute medication is being taken, particularly where there is potential for medication overuse headache.
- When acute medication is intolerable or ineffective.
- In special circumstances such as hemiplegic migraine where there can be risk of permanent neurological injury.
- Patient attitudes towards taking medication on a regular basis.

Episodic preventive treatment

It is used when there is a known headache trigger. For example, indometacin for the prevention of exercise-induced migraine.

Short-term prevention

This is used when the problem is time limited. For example, menstrual migraine.

Long-term prevention

- Consider patient preference.
- Establish co-morbidity for treatment preferences or avoidance.
- Establish plans or potential risk of pregnancy.
- Start at a low dose and increase slowly to the maximum recommended dose or when side effects become problematic (migraineurs are often more sensitive to medication and their side effects).
- Continue for at least 6 weeks on the maximum dose that can be tolerated before judging effectiveness.
- Give the patient clear written instructions and advise of main side effects.
- Length of therapy. Discuss discontinuation at 6 months with patient and reduce drug slowly if stopping.
  - Migraine headache may improve independently of treatment
  - Successful treatment may allow patient to readjust their life style with beneficial effects
  - Successful treatment may 'turn off' the migraine process

Medication options

Choice of drug will depend on co-morbidity, patient preference and setting. The evidence base is of variable quality and, in many cases, clinical impression predominates. With the exception of methylsergide, all preventative drugs have been found to be of use serendipitously. Many are not licensed despite widespread use, and this fact should be discussed with the patient (see Chapter 1).

From the perspective of primary care, a reasonable approach would be:
- β-Blocker
- Amitriptyline particularly if there is co-existent anxiety, poor sleep or depression.
- Pizotifen. Commonly used in primary care but limited effectiveness and troublesome weight gain.
- Anticonvulsants

Below are shown the options and relative indications. Of the drugs listed, only propranolol, metoprolol, timolol, nadolol pizotifen, topiramate and methysergide have a licence for migraine in the UK.

This information is for guidance only. Prescribers should read manufacturer's product information details or refer to the *British National Formulary* for further information.

β-Blockers

The mode of action is not known. There are probably no differences between the β-blockers in terms of efficacy although if one doesn't works it may be worth trying another. Atenolol is a reasonable first choice as it is once a day, cheap and relatively side effect free. Nebivolol is a useful alternative if side effects are problematic.

Drugs	Think about using	Caution	Side effects
Atenolol—25–100mg			
Propranolol—20mg tds increasing to 40mg tds—useful if there is underlying anxiety	Hypertension, angina, cardiac failure	Asthma, depression, Raynaud's disease, diabetes. Unstable, heart failure. Don't use with verapamil, reduce dose of rizatriptan with propranolol, hypotensive effect agonized by steroids	Bradycardia, hypotension, peripheral vasoconstriction, bronchospasm, fatigue, sexual dysfunction. Enhanced hypotensive effect
Nebivolol 2.5—5mg relatively low side effect profile			

Antidepressants

Mode of action not known. Particularly useful with co-morbid depression. Only amitriptyline has demonstrated benefits and is useful with anxiety or poor sleep. No evidence for SSRIs, but are used in practice. SSRIs and TCAs can be given together. Antihistamine and anticholinergic properties limit the use of TCAs.

Drug	Think about using	Caution	Side effects
Amitriptyline— start at a low dose 5–10mg. If troublesome side effects try nortriptyline or dosulepin	Other co-morbid painful disorders, depression, anxiety, insomnia	Heart block, urinary retention, epilepsy (lowers convulsive threshold), drugs—alcohol increases sedative effect, plasma concentration increased with antipsychotics	Dry mouth, sedation, blurred vision, constipation, difficulty with micturition, arrhythmias, syncope, confusion, increased appetite
SSRIs—fluoxetine 20mg; citalopram 20–40mg		Epilepsy, cardiac disease, susceptibility to angle closure glaucoma. Triptans theoretically increase serotonergic effects, but in practice the risks are small (see Chapter 4)	Gastrointestinal effects similar to TCAs but less severe

Anticonvulsants

Migraine and epilepsy share similar features and there may be similar mechanisms in their action. Topiramate is the only licensed drug.

Drug	Think about using	Caution	Side effects
Topiramate—initially 25mg a day increasing by 25mg each week to a maximum of 50mg bd	Co-morbid epilepsy	Ensure adequate hydration especially if predisposition to nephrolithiasis. Avoid if porphyria, hepatic or renal impairment. Can exacerbate or precipitate depression	Paraesthesia, cognitive impairment, nausea, abdominal pain, dyspepsia, weight loss, taste disturbance, speech disorder, depression. Suicidal ideation can occur

Drug	Think about using	Caution	Side effects
Sodium valproate—initially 200mg bd increasing to maximum of 600mg bd. Most patients achieve benefit from 300mg bd. Few will gain benefit from higher doses. Modified release tablets have theoretical advantages		SLE, liver disease, porphyrea, hepatic dysfunction. Check baseline LFTs and once during first 6 months	Hair loss, sedation, tremor, cognitive impairments, nausea, vomiting, dyspepsia. Has been associated with acute closure glaucoma
Gabapentin—300mg on day 1 increasing to 300mg bd/tds each day. Maximum 1.8g/day	Anxiety disorders	History of psychotic illness, renal impairment	Gastrointestinal problems, ataxia, paraesthesia, dysarthria

5-HT receptor antagonists

Cyproheptadine is similar to pizotifen but not used in the UK. Methysergide is an ergot alkaloid and should be used under specialist supervision. It is useful for refractory migraine when other agents have failed.

Drug	Think about using	Caution	Side effects
Pizotifen—1.5mg at night time increasing to a single dose of 3mg at night or 1.5mg during the day and 3mg at night	More effective in children. Limited effectiveness in adults	Urinary retention, angle closure glaucoma, renal impairment	Weight gain, drowsiness

Drug	Think about using	Caution	Side effects
Methysergide—start with a 1mg a day and increase by 1mg every 2–3 days to a maximum of 2mg tds	In refractory migraine, orthostatic hypotension. Specialist initiation only due to side effects	Ischaemic heart disease, peripheral vascular disease, lung disease, collagen disease, valve and heart disease. Avoid erythromycin or other ergot alkaloids. Increased peripheral vasoconstriction with β-blockers, increased risk of vasospasm with triptans	Nausea, vomiting, diarrhoea, dyspepsia, hallucinations. The major complication (1 in 2000) is retroperitoneal, pulmendocardial fibrosis. To minimize fibrosis, give it 6 months and then have a 1-month drug holiday phasing out drug over a 1-week period. Long-term therapy may need regular echocardiogram, chest X-ray and abdominal MRI

Calcium channel blockers

These regulate a number of membrane mechanisms affecting the release or entry at calcium channels. Only flunarizine is supported by consistent evidence. Flunarizine doesn't have a UK licence but is in widespread use in Europe.

Drug	Think about using	Caution	Side effects
Flunarizine—5mg increasing to 10mg at night after 1 month	Hypertension, familial hemiplegic migraine	Parkinson disease	Tiredness, weight gain, depression
Verapamil—80mg bd increasing to a maximum of 240mg bd	Migraine with aura, hypertension, ischaemic heart disease	First degree AV block, myocardial infarct, hepatic impairment. Avoid grapefruit juice. Avoid with β-blockers and other antiarrhythmics. Metabolism inhibited by clarithromycin and erythromycin with increased risk of toxicity. Antifungals can give increased plasma concentration. Enhanced hypotensive effect with antipsychotics	Constipation, hypotension

Non-steroidal anti-inflammatories

Evidence exists for aspirin and naproxen.

Drug	Think about using	Caution	Side effects
Aspirin 300mg bd; naproxen 500mg bd	With other inflammatory conditions	Dyspepsia, past history of peptic ulcer. Asthma, coagulation defects, renal impairment, severe heart failure	Gastrointestinal disorder, provocation of renal failure, elevation of blood pressure, fluid retention

Other drugs

Limited evidence exists for a number of other drugs that are in clinic use. Some may be useful if co-morbidities are present. All are unlicensed.

Drug	Think about using	Caution	Side effects
ACE inhibitors: lisinopril—10–20mg od	Hypertension, cardiac failure	Patients receiving diuretics, athersclerosis, renal impairment and renal artery stenosis	Hypotension, renal impairment, cough
Angiotensin II antagonist: candesartan—8mg increasing to maximum of 32mg	As above	As above	Less cough. vertigo
Clonidine— 50-75mcg bd	Often used in primary care but ineffective	No place in the management of migraine	

Non-pharmaceutical alternative preventative medication

There is Grade B evidence for the following compounds. There may be problems with standardization and purity

Drug	Notes
Feverfew (dried chrysanthemum leaves)	6.25mg tds. Side effects include abdominal pain and soreness of the oral mucosa
Butterbur (obtained from a perennial shrub)	50-75mg bd. No side effects noted
Magnesium salts	600mg$^+$ Diarrhoea is the main problem. Dicitrate has less laxative effects than hydroxide, oxide and sulphate. Low magnesium has been noted in the brains of migraine sufferers. 3 months may be needed to evalulate for benefit
Riboflavin (water-soluble vitamin)	Acts on the mitochondrial electron transport chain. 400mg a day (cf. dietary requirement of 4.5mg per day). Diarrhoea is the main side effect
Co-enzyme Q10	Acts at mitochondrial level as riboflavin. Used in a wide range of other conditions. No noted side effects. 100mg tds

Occipital nerve manipulation

The second order neurons from C1 and C2 spinal afferents converge upon the trigeminal nucleus caudalis and dorsal horn nuclei which are implicated in the pathogenesis of headache. Manipulation of occipital nerve afferents offers opportunities to modulate the dynamics of this area with possible therapeutic benefit.

Occipital nerve injection

- Occipital nerve zone tenderness is clinically associated with headache syndromes.
- Injection of this nerve has been used for a range of headaches including cervicogenic headache, occipital neuralgia, migraine and cluster headache.
- The response rate is ~50%, with a greater efficacy in those who demonstrate tenderness over the occipital nerve.
- The response may take up to 2 days.
- The duration of complete response can range from 1 day to 3 months and is less for cluster than migraine.
- Analgesia or triptan overuse does not affect response.
- Adverse effects are infrequent and can include:
  - Transient dizziness
  - Alopecia around the site of injection
  - Headaches triggered or exacerbated following the injection
- This technique is useful
  - To provide interim relief while other approaches are explored
  - In pregnancy when other options are limited
- Rigorous trials of efficacy are awaited.

Occipital nerve stimulation (ONS)

- Subcutaneous and epidural neurostimulation approaches have been used for a number of years in the treatment of peripheral pain syndromes.
- Based on experimental findings of convergence of trigeminal and occipital inputs onto second order trigeminocervical neurons and human functional imaging evidence for changes in brain activation in chronic migraine with headache relief during ONS, this potential therapy is being studied.
- Studies in chronic migraine are ongoing, comparing active and sham stimuli and the results are expected in 2009.
- ONS has been reported to be useful in medically intractable chronic cluster headache and hemicrania continua, and certainly deserves more intensive evaluation.
- ONS does remain a treatment of last resort, requiring more clinical trial data, and its use is limited to carefully supervised patients in experienced centres or in clinical trial settings.

Table 5.12 Practical guidance for occipital nerve injection

- Identify the occipital nerve. This lies in the occipital groove which is approximately mid-way along the occipital ridge between the occipital tubercle and mastoid process. Invariably the patient will be tender at this point.
- Inject 80mg methylprednisolone and 1ml 2% lidocaine. If both sides are tender, 40mg methylprednisolone is injected into each side. Otherwise 80mg into the one side.
- A blue needle is inserted above the occipital groove and the mixture injected in a fan shape ~1cm arch as shown in the diagram.
- A suitable consent form is given in Appendix 4.

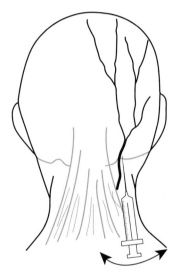

Fig. 5.3 Injection of the occipital nerve.

Migraine in women

Migraine and menstruation

Around 25% of women experience migraine at some point during their lives. At least 50% of women with migraine report an association between migraine attacks and menstruation.

Clinical features

- For most women with menstrual attacks, migraine also occurs at other times of the month ('menstrually related' migraine).
- 10% of women report migraine exclusively with menstruation and at no other time of the month ('pure' menstrual migraine) (see Table 6.1).
- A few women report a constant association between migraine and menstruation since menarche.
- Most women report a gradual association between migraine and menstruation developing from their late 30s, with increasing prevalence in the years leading to menopause.
- Following the menopause, migraine prevalence declines.
- Migraine is most likely to occur on or between 2 days before menstruation and the first 3 days of bleeding (see Fig. 6.2).
- Menstrual attacks are almost invariably *without* aura, even in women who have attacks *with* aura at other times of the cycle.
- Attacks occurring at the time of menstruation are more severe and disabling, last longer and are less responsive to symptomatic medication (see Table 6.2).

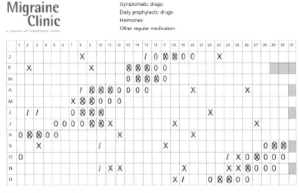

Fig. 6.1 A diary card to assess menstrual migraine.
X = Migraine. **/** = Headache. **0** = Period

Table 6.1 IHS diagnostic criteria for pure menstrual migraine and menstrually related migraine without aura

---

Pure menstrual migraine without aura

Diagnostic criteria:

A. Attacks, in a menstruating woman, fulfilling criteria for migraine without aura

B. Attacks occur exclusively on day (i.e, days −2 to +3) of menstruation in at least two out of three menstrual cycles and at no other times of the cycle

Menstrually related migraine without aura

Diagnostic criteria:

A. Attacks, in a menstruating woman, fulfilling criteria for migraine without aura

B. Attacks occur on day 1±2 (i.e, days −2 to +3) of menstruation in at least two out of three menstrual cycles and additionally at other times of the cycle

---

The first day of menstruation is day 1 and the preceding day is day −1; there is no day 0. For the purposes of this classification, menstruation is considered to be endometrial bleeding resulting from either the normal menstrual cycle or from the withdrawal of exogenous progestogens, as in the case of combined oral contraceptives and cyclical hormone replacement therapy

Pathophysiology

- Studies have not identified any consistent biochemical or hormonal abnormalities in women with menstrual migraine, compared with control groups.
- The most likely mechanism to account for perimenstrual migraine is falling levels of oestrogen following prolonged oestrogen exposure, such as occurs during the late luteal phase of the normal menstrual cycle (see Fig 6.2).
- Migraine associated with menorrhagia and/or dysmenorrhoea may be associated with prostaglandins and prostaglandin metabolites in the systemic circulation, which occurs during the first 48h of menstruation.
- Hormone fluctuations associated with the perimenopause may account for increased prevalence of menstrual migraine in this group of women.

Diagnosis

- Confirm the diagnosis using diary cards (Fig. 6.1) to record migraine and menstruation over a minimum of three consecutive cycles.

Investigations

- There are no investigations to confirm or refute the diagnosis of menstrual migraine

Treatment

- Management strategies are outlined in Fig. 6.3.
- There are no drugs licensed for the treatment of menstrual migraine in the UK at the time of writing—all drugs must be prescribed off-licence,
- It is sensible to try a method for at least three cycles before considering alternative prophylaxis.
- Optimize symptomatic treatment, which may suffice without need of further intervention,
- Consider prophylaxis if response to symptomatic treatment for migraine attacks is inadequate,
- Review regularly, with diary cards, every 3–6 cycles until migraine is stabilized.
- Although many women favour non-drug approaches, these appear to be ineffective for menstrual migraine

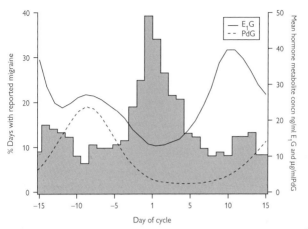

Fig 6.2 Incidence of migraine, urinary oestrone-3-glucuronide (E₁G) and pregnane-diol-3-glucuronide (PdG) levels on each day of the menstrual cycle in 120 cycles from 38 women. Reproduced with permission from MacGregor EA, et al. (2006). Prevalence of migraine on each day of the natural menstrual cycle. *Neurology*. **67**: 2154–8.

Table 6.2 Relative risk of severe migraine at menstruation

Day around onset of menses	Odds ratio of severe migraine (confidence intervals)	Significance level
−5 to −1	1.43 (1.00–2.00)	0.05
−2 to −1	2.06 (1.29–3.13)	0.003
+1 to +3	3.41 (2.58–4.47)	<0.0001
+1 to +6	2.63 (2.07–3.35)	<0.0001

Based on MacGregor EA, et al. (2004). Prevalence of migraine on each day of the natural menstrual cycle. *Neurology*. **63**(2): 351–3.

Non-steroidal anti-inflammatory drugs

- NSAIDs should be tried as first-line agents for migraine attacks that start on the first to third day of bleeding, particularly in the presence of dysmenorrhoea and/or menorrhagia
  - Mefenamic acid 500mg 3–4 times daily
  - Start 2–3 days before the expected onset of menstruation and continue for the first 2–3 days of bleeding
  - If periods are irregular start on the first day of bleeding
  - Naproxen 500mg once or twice daily is an alternative.
- Side effects of NSAIDs include gastrointestinal disturbance.
- Contraindications include peptic ulcer and aspirin-induced allergy.
- Interactions include anticoagulants and antihypertensive agents.

Perimenstrual oestrogen supplements

- Estradiol gel 1.5mg applied once daily from 2–3 days before expected menstruation for 7 days.
- An alternative is transdermal oestrogen 100mcg from 2–3 days before expected menstruation up to the fourth or fifth day of menstruation.
- Some women responding to oestrogen supplements experience delayed attacks when the supplements are discontinued. The duration of supplement use can be extended until day 7 of the cycle, tapering the dose by halving it over each of the last 2 days.
- Oestrogen supplements can be used only when menstruation is regular and predictable.
- No additional progestogens are necessary, provided that the woman is ovulating regularly.
- Ovulation can be confirmed using a home-use fertility monitor, which has the advantage of predicting menstruation.
- There is no evidence of increased risk of thrombosis or cancer in women already producing endogenous oestrogen. Supplemental oestrogens are not recommended for women who have oestrogen-dependent tumours or other oestrogen-dependent conditions, including a history of venous thromboembolism.

Perimenstrual triptans

- Trials using frovatriptan, naratriptan, sumatriptan and zolmitriptan for perimenstrual prophylaxis have suggested efficacy.
- Perimenstrual triptans should be considered for women with menstrual migraine in whom standard strategies fail.
- Frovatriptan has undergone extensive clinical trials using the following 6-day regime
  - Start perimenstrual prophylaxis 2 days before the expected menstrual attack
  - On the first day of treatment take 5mg frovatriptan twice daily

Continue frovatriptan 2.5mg twice daily for a further 5 days.

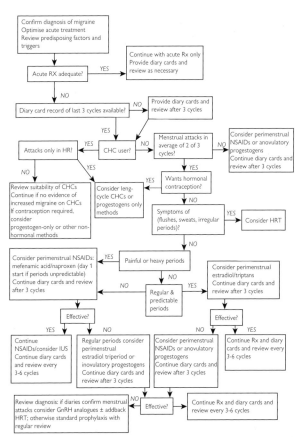

Fig. 6.3 Algorithm for the management of menstrual attacks of migraine. CHC = combined hormonal contraceptives; GnRH = gonadotrophin-releasing hormone; HFI = hormone-free interval; HRT = hormone replacement therapy; IUS = intra-uterine system; NSAIDs = non-steroidal anti-inflammatory drugs. Reproduced with permission from MacGregor EA, *et al.* (2007). Menstrual migraine: a clinical review. *J Fam Plann Reprod Health Care.* **33**(1): 36-47.

Other strategies to consider
Hormonal contraceptives
- Women who also require contraception may benefit from contraceptives that eliminate the ovarian cycle (see below).

Gonadotrophin-releasing hormone analogues
- GnRH analogues have been shown to be effective in clinical trials.
- Adverse effects of oestrogen deficiency, e.g. hot flushes, restrict their use.
- Treatment is associated with a marked reduction in bone density and should not usually be used for longer than 6 months without regular monitoring and bone densitometry.
- 'Add-back' continuous combined oestrogen and progestogen can be given to counter these difficulties.
- Given these limitations, in addition to cost, such treatment should be instigated only in specialist departments, but is worth considering if all other options fail.

Migraine and the menopause
- The natural history of migraine is to diminish with increasing age.
- For women who experience menstrual migraine then the problem is likely to get worse perimenopausally with fluctuating oestrogen levels.
- Migraine is more likely to deteriorate after surgical menopause with bilateral oophorectomy.
- Hormone replacement treatment is the treatment of choice particularly when migraine is accompanied by other perimenopausal symptoms.
- Both oestrogen and progestogen can exacerbate migraine if not optimized. Treatment can be difficult as some women can develop headaches as a result of the therapy (see Table 6.3). If migraine persists once other menopause symptoms are controlled, review non-hormonal triggers and management strategies.

Table 6.3 Hormone replacement treatment of perimenopausal migraine

- Use a continuous non-oral form of oestrogen replacement.
- Start with a low dose which can gradually be increased. Too much oestrogen given too quickly can exacerbate migraine. For example, use a 25mcg estradiol matrix patch. The optimal dose is the dose that controls hot flushes.
- Switch to tibolone if unsuccessful.
- Progestogen should be given to protect endometrium but can also exacerbate migraine.
  - Switch from a cyclical to a continuous lower dose progestogen, e.g. continuous patch combined with oestrogen
  - Change progestogen type

Migraine and contraception

For the majority of women including those with migraine, combined hormonal contraceptives (CHCs) are a highly effective and safe means of contraception with added health benefits. However, for a minority of women with specific risk factors, including migraine with aura, CHCs are associated with added health risks.

Effect of CHCs on headache and migraine

- Compared with baseline, headache increases during the early cycles of CHC use but improves with continued use.
- Women experiencing headache in the first cycle of CHCs have only a 1 in 3 chance of experiencing headache in the 2nd cycle and a 1 in 10 chance in the 3rd cycle.
- Women aged ≥35, and those with a strong personal or family history of headaches, are more likely to report worsening or new onset of headache associated with CHCs.
- Neither the dose of ethinylestradiol nor the dose or type of progestogen appear to influence headache or migraine.

Effect of CHCs on migraine with aura

- Migraine with aura is more likely to worsen following CHC use and may appear for the first time.
- Use of CHCs is associated with a 1.5- to 2-fold increased risk of ischaemic stroke.
- Other independent risk factors for ischaemic stroke include:
  - Smoking
  - Hypertension
  - Migraine with aura (see Table 6.4).
- Pre-existing migraine with aura is considered a contraindication to CHCs by most authorities (see Table 6.5).
- Women developing migraine aura associated with CHCs should immediately switch to a progestogen-only or non-hormonal method of contraception.
- Contraceptive efficacy is not affected as other methods are as effective, or more effective than CHCs (see Table 6.6).

Migraine in the hormone-free interval

- Headache and migraine without aura related to CHC use are most likely to occur during the hormone-free interval, typically around the third day (see Fig 6.2d).
- The mechanism is typically oestrogen 'withdrawal'.
- Changing from a 30-35 mcg ethinylestradiol method to a 20 mcg method has minimal effect given that all low-dose CHCs substantially elevate oestrogen levels above normal levels.

Table 6.4 Risk of ischaemic stroke in CHC users

	Odds ratio of migraine without aura (95%CI)	Odds ratio of migraine with aura (95%CI)
Tzourio et al. (1995)	3.0 (1.5–5.8)	6.2 (2.1–18.0)
Carolei et al. (1996)	1.0 (0.5–2.0)	8.6 (1–75)
Chang et al. (1999)	3.0 (0.7–13.5)	3.8 (1.3–11.5)

Table 6.5 Recommendations for use of CHCs in women with migraine with aura

Pre-existing migraine with aura
Contraceptive use of CHCs contraindicated by some authorities

New-onset aura after starting CHCs
Stop CHCs and provide emergency contraception if necessary and progestogen-only or non-hormonal method of contraception

>5 years past (but not current) headache with aura
CHCs possible with counselling and warning to stop immediately if aura develops

Table 6.6 Method failure rates per 100 woman years

Methods	Failure rate per 100 women years	
	Perfect use	Typical use
COC	0.1	3
POP	0.5	5
Desogesterol	0.1	0.4
Levonorgestrel IUS	0.1	0.1
Medroxyprogesterone acetate (Depo-Provera)	0.3	3
Etonogestrel (Implanon)	0.05	0.05
T380 IUD	0.6	0.8
Female sterilization	0.5	0.5

- Effective methods to control headaches in the hormone-free interval include:
  - 100mcg oestrogen patches: first patch on day 21; replace with new patch on day 24 or 25 (3rd/4th day of hormone-free interval); remove on 1st day of next CHC pack.
  - Oestrogen supplements
  - Long-cycle CHCs, i.e. running 3–4 packs together back to back before a 7-day break
  - Continuous CHCs, i.e. continuous use of CHCs without a break.
- There is increasing evidence of the benefits, safety and efficacy of continuous combined CHCs.
- Breakthrough bleeding can occur with continuous CHCs, but this typically resolves with continued use.

Effect of progestogen-only methods on migraine

Few studies differentiate between headache and migraine, most citing incidence of headache only. Consequently, adverse events reporting headache will include migraine. Progestogen-only contraception does not have any adverse effects on thrombotic parameters, and use of these methods is not associated with an increased risk of ischaemic stroke. Hence, they are a safe and effective alternative for women for whom oestrogen-containing methods are contraindicated.

Progestogen-only pill

Improvement is more likely in women who become amenorrhoeic, It may be necessary to double the dose (off-licence) to achieve this.

Subdermal implants

Retrospective non-comparative studies suggest that the reported incidence of headache is not increased among women using subdermal implants such as Implanon.

Depot progestogens

- Studies suggest that there are no significant changes in headache from baseline in women using depot medoxyprogesterone actetate (DMPA).
- Anecdotally, headache can occur with breakthrough bleeding in early cycles of use and typically resolves once amenorrhoea is achieved.

Levonorgestrel intrauterine system

- Headache is a common complaint in early months of use.
- Reported as a significant reason for removal compared with women using copper IUs ((1.9% vs 0.25% at 5 years).
- There is evidence that headache occurring in the early months of use can settle with continued use.

Effect of non-hormonal methods on migraine

- Headache is reported as an adverse event in trials of non-hormonal methods, which is not surprising since headache and migraine is a common complaint in all women.
- Anecdotally, 'menstrual' headache is more common in women with dysmenorrhoea and menorrhagia, which occur in association with copper IUDs.

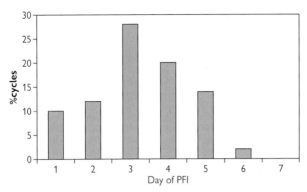

Fig. 6.4 Incidence of migraine on each day of the pill-free interval (PFI). Unpublished data from MacGregor (2002).

Migraine and pregnancy

The majority of women with pre-existing migraine improve during pregnancy. Drugs and other teratogens exert their greatest effects on the foetus in the first trimester. Women planning a pregnancy would benefit from having their medication reviewed and, if necessary changed to a safer alternative in the lowest effective dose. Frequent pre-pregnancy headache is a strong predictor of poor general and emotional health during pregnancy—assess for depressive disorders.

Clinical features

Effect of pregnancy on migraine

- 60–70% of women with pre-existing migraine improve during pregnancy
  - 20% of attacks completely resolve during pregnancy
  - Improvement is more likely if pre-existing migraine is without aura, particularly if attacks are related to menstruation.
- If migraine has not improved by the end of the 1st trimester, it is likely to continue throughout pregnancy. Improvement is less likely if pre-existing migraine is with aura.
- Aura may develop for the first time in pregnancy.
- First ever migraine during pregnancy is more likely to be with aura.

Effect of migraine on pregnancy

- There is no evidence that migraine with or without aura has any adverse effect of pregnancy outcome in otherwise healthy women.
- Increased risk of pre-eclampsia and eclampsia in women with migraine, particularly in overweight women

Postpartum

- 30–40% of women experience headache in the week following delivery.
- Risk of cerebral infarction is increased during 6 weeks post-partum.
- Risk is increased in women with history of migraine, pre-eclampsia and gestational hypertension .
- Breastfeeding should be encouraged and is associated with less migraine compared with women who bottle-feed.
- Return of menstruation is associated with increased migraine.

Investigation

Consider investigating first ever migraine in pregnancy (see Tables 6.7 and 6.8).

Table 6.7 Disorders in pregnancy that can be associated with aura and/or headache

- Thrombocytopenia
- Cerebral venous sinus thrombosis
- Eclampsia
- Stroke
- Subarachnoid haemorrhage
- Pituitary tumour
- Choriocarcinoma

Table 6.8 Investigating headache

- Investigate suspected secondary headache
- Investigations are the same as for non-pregnant women
- Radiological testing should not be deferred purely on account of pregnancy
- Use MRI if possible
- Head CT is relatively safe for possible acute bleeds

Treatment

Identification of non-hormonal triggers

- Non-hormonal migraine triggers should be identified and eliminated where possible.
- Women should be encouraged to
  - Avoid missed meals
  - Take regular exercise
  - Drink plenty of fluids
  - Maintain a regular sleep pattern.

Drugs in pregnancy and lactation

- Few drugs have been tested for safety during pregnancy and lactation; evidence of safety is usually circumstantial, therefore most drugs use is unlicensed.
- Drugs should only be used if the potential benefits outweigh risks to the foetus.
- When recommending use of a drug in contradiction to the prescribing information in the Summary of Product Characteristics, the risks and benefits should be discussed with the woman, who may choose to use the drug on a named patient basis.
- The discussion should be documented in the notes.

Symptomatic treatment during pregnancy

- Analgesics and antiemetics commonly used for the treatment of migraine can be continued throughout pregnancy.
- NSAIDs, including aspirin and ibuprofen, can be taken in the 1st and 2nd trimesters, but should be avoided near term.
- Although a positive recommendation to use triptans during pregnancy cannot be made on the limited data available, women who have taken triptans can be reassured that their use is highly unlikely to result in any adverse outcome.
- Ergots are contraindicated.
- If there are no other risk factors involved, inadvertent exposure to any of the drugs used for the treatment of migraine, even those contraindicated for use during pregnancy, does not constitute medical grounds for termination of pregnancy.

Symptomatic treatment during lactation

- An appropriate strategy is
  - Diclofenac 50-100mg PO or PR, up to 200mg per 24h,
  - Combined with domperidone 20mg PO or 30–60mg PR up to 4 doses per 24h.
- Sumatriptan can be used during breastfeeding.
- There is little reason why other triptans with low bioavailability and low absorption by the infant such as eletriptan, naratriptan, rizatriptan or zolmitriptan should not also be used.
- Even minor exposure could be largely avoided by expressing and discarding all milk for ~4h after dosing.

Table 6.9 Symptomatic drugs: use during pregnancy and lactation

	1st trimester	2nd trimester	3rd trimester	Lactation
Acetaminophen/ paracetamol	✓	✓	✓	✓
Codeine	(✓)	(✓)	(✓)	✓
Aspirin	(✓)	(✓)	Avoid	Avoid
Diclofenac	(✓)	(✓)	Avoid	✓
Ibuprofen	(✓)	(✓)	Avoid	✓
Naproxen	(✓)	(✓)	Avoid	✓
Buclizine	(✓)	(✓)	(✓)	✓
Cyclizine	(✓)	(✓)	(✓)	✓
Domperidone	(✓)	(✓)	(✓)	✓
Doxylamine	(✓)	(✓)	(✓)	(✓)
Metoclopramide	(✓)	(✓)	(✓)	(✓)
Prochlorperazine*	(✓)	(✓)	(✓)	✓
Dihydroergotamine	C/I	C/I	C/I	Avoid
Ergotamine	C/I	C/I	C/I	Avoid
Almotriptan	ID	ID	ID	W
Eletriptan	ID	ID	ID	W
Frovatriptan	ID	ID	ID	W
Naratriptan	?(✓)	?(✓)	?(✓)	(✓)
Rizatriptan	?(✓)	?(✓)	?(✓)	W
Sumatriptan	?(✓)	?(✓)	?(✓)	W
Zolmitriptan	ID	ID	ID	(✓)
Chlorpromazine IM*	(✓)	(✓)	(✓)	✓
Magnesium sulphate IV*	(✓)	(✓)	(✓)	(✓)
Prednisolone*	(✓)	(✓)	(✓)	(✓)

C/I = contraindicated; ID = insufficient data; ?(✓) = limited data but probably safe; (✓) = data suggest unlikely to cause harm; ✓ = no evidence of harm. W = withhold breastfeeding for 12–24 hours after dosing

*Emergency treatment of migraine not responding to standard measures.

Reproduced with permission from MacGregor EA, et al. (2007). Menstrual migraine: a clinical review. *J Fam Plann Reprod Health Care*. **33**(1): 36-47.

Specific prophylaxis for migraine in pregnancy and lactation

Non-drug prophylaxis
- Relaxation, biofeedback and physical therapy are safe and effective treatment alternatives for 80% of pregnant women.
- Benefits are maintained beyond pregnancy

Drug prophylaxis in pregnancy
- Consider the natural history of improvement during the 2nd and 3rd trimesters before instigating drug prophylaxis
- The recommended prophylactic is propranolol. This drug has been widely used and there is no indication of an increased risk of malformations when it is used for migraine prevention during pregnancy.
  - Ideally, the lowest effective dose should be used, starting with 10–20mg bd.
  - Propranolol should be stopped 2–3 days before delivery in order to reduce the occurrence of slowed heart rate in the baby and a reduction in uterine contractions.
  - Consider monitoring the baby for hypoglycaemia.
- *Amitriptyline* 10–50mg at night can be used throughout pregnancy.
- A further alternative is topiramate in the lowest effective dose.

Drug prophylaxis in lactation
Propranolol in doses of 10-20mg twice daily is a first-line strategy.

Failure of treatment response
- Review the diagnosis, as this is the most likely reason for ineffective management.
- Medication overuse headache can also present during pregnancy, and should be considered in any woman regularly taking symptomatic treatments for headache on >3 days a week, every week.

Emergency treatment during pregnancy
- IM prochlorperazine 10mg or chlorpromazine 25–50mg together with IV fluids.
- IV magnesium sulphate 1g 12hrly.
- Intravenous prochlorperazine 10mg 8hrly together with IV magnesium sulphate 1g 12hrly for prolonged aura.

Further information
The National Teratology Information Service (NTIS)
Regional Drug & Therapeutics Centre,
Wolfson Unit,
Claremont Place,
Newcastle upon Tyne NE2 4HH
Mon-Fri Tel: 0191 232 1525 Fax: 0191 260 6193 (office hours)
Tel. 0191 282 5944 (urgent enquiries, 17:00–20:00 Monday to Friday)

The NTIS is funded by the Department of Health to provide a national service on all aspects of toxicity of drugs and chemicals in pregnancy throughout the UK.

Table 6.10 Prophylactic drugs for use during pregnancy and lactation

	1st trimester	2nd trimester	3rd trimester	Lactation
Amitriptyline	(✓)	(✓)	(✓)	(✓)
Low-dose aspirin	(✓)	(✓)	Avoid	Avoid
Atenolol	Avoid	Avoid	Avoid	(✓)
Gabapentin	ID	?(✓)	?(✓)	ID
Methysergide	C/I	C/I	C/I	C/I
Metoprolol	(✓)	(✓)	(✓)	✓
Pizotifen	ID	ID	ID	ID
Propranolol	(✓)	(✓)	(✓)	✓
Topiramate	ID	(✓)	(✓)	ID
Valproate	C/I	ID	C/I	✓
Verapamil	(✓)	(✓)	avoid	✓

C/I = contraindicated; ID = insufficient data; ?(✓) = limited data but probably safe; (✓) = data suggest unlikely to cause harm; ✓ = no evidence of harm.

Table 6.11 Herbs/vitamins for migraine to use during pregnancy and lactation

	1st trimester	2nd trimester	3rd trimester	Lactation
Vitamin B2 (riboflavin)	✓*	✓*	✓*	✓*
Vitamin B6 (pyridoxine)	✓*	✓*	✓*	✓*
Coenzyme Q10	ID	ID	ID	✓*
Feverfew	C/I	C/I	C/I	CI
Butterbur	ID	ID	ID	ID
Ginger	(✓)*	(✓)*	(✓)*	(✓)*

C/I = contraindicated; ID = insufficient data; ?(✓) = limited data but probably safe; (✓) = data suggest unlikely to cause harm; ✓ = no evidence of harm.

*Avoid mega doses

Reproduced with permission from MacGregor EA, et al. (2007). Menstrual migraine: a clinical review. *J Fam Plann Reprod Health Care*. **33**(1): 36-47.

Tension-type headache

Introduction

Tension-type headache (TTH) is a frequently diagnosed yet poorly understood condition. It is generally regarded as a 'featureless', bilateral headache that is never severe and does not limit physical activity.

A variety of names have been applied to this disorder, including 'tension headache', 'muscle contraction headache', 'psychogenic headache', 'ordinary headache', 'psychomyogenic headache' and 'stress headache'. The use of the term tension does not imply that the patient is suffering from mental tension or stress.

In clinical practice, one is generally aiming to:
- Exclude underlying potential serious pathology.
- Identify features that allow an alternative diagnosis of migraine to be made.

Classification

IHS classifications are shown in Table 7.1. Three types are identified:
- Infrequent
- Frequent
- Chronic

From a clinical perspective:
- Current classifications are defined to facilitate research into headache disorders and often have limitations in the clinic setting.
- The main area of controversy is whether features that are generally regarded as 'migrainous' in the diagnosis (e.g. photophobia, phonophobia, nausea) should be allowed.
- Diagnostic difficulties will arise if diagnosis is made on the basis of exclusion rather than inclusion of features.
- In practice, a diagnosis of TTH should only be made by taking a detailed and thorough history.

Table 7.1 IHS classification of headache

Clinical characteristics:
- At least three of the following pain characteristics:
  - Bilateral location
  - Pressing/tightening (non-pulsatile) quality
  - Mild or moderate intensity
  - Not aggravated by routine activity such as walking or climbing stairs
- No nausea (anorexia may occur), vomiting, photophobia or phonophobia
- Not attributed to another disorder

TTH classifications:
- Infrequent episodic TTH. At least 10 episodes occurring on <1 day per month on average (<12 days/year).
- Frequent episodic TTH. At least 10 episodes occurring on ≥1 but <15 days/ month for at least 3 months (≥12 and <180 days/year).
- Chronic TTH. Headache occurring on ≥15 days/month on average for >3 months (≥180 days/year)

Clinical features

In general, the pain of TTH is:

- Dull, aching and non-pulsatile feeling of tightness, pressure or constriction that may be band-like or patchy.
- It commonly spreads to the occiput and down into the neck, but location varies between individuals and it can affect any part of the cranium.
- It may or may not be associated with a degree of pericranial or neck muscle tenderness.
- Pain may last for hours or even days, and is usually bearable.
- The fundamental difference between TTH and migraine is that TTH lacks features of sensory sensitivity of any description, so absolutely no nausea and no sensitivity to light, sound or smell should be allowed. It never throbs and is not aggravated by routine physical activity.
- Episodic TTH has low impact and is usually managed satisfactorily by the patient.
- Chronic TTH can have significant impact on quality of life and socio-economic cost.
- Features raising the possibility of, or indicating, an alternative diagnosis of migraine should be pursued (see Table 7.2).

Differential diagnosis

- The important differential diagnosis is secondary headache due to underlying pathology. In particular:
  - Tumour
  - Giant cell arteritis
  - High and low pressure syndromes
- One condition that is often misdiagnosed as chronic TTH is new daily persistent headache.
  - Featureless bilateral pressure or constricting headaches.
  - Patient will typically recall the actual day of onset of a headache that arrived out of the blue and persisted on a regular daily basis.

Tension-type headache and migraine

TTH may be part of a migraine spectrum.

- Factor analysis studies fail to find clinical features that distinguish the two conditions.
- The majority of migraineurs also have TTH.
- Approximately 25% of TTH patients have migraine.
- Migraine may also cause pericranial muscle tenderness.
- Routine physical activity exacerbates TTH in those patients who also have migraine.
- Photophobia, phonophobia, and nausea are more frequent in TTH where there is co-morbid migraine.
- Migraineurs may experience TTH triggered by alcohol, cheese, chocolate and exertion.
- The early phase of migraine may resemble TTH, and patient reporting may be distorted by use of acute attack medication.
- Triptans abort TTH in patients with frequent migraine.
- Both conditions are associated with:
  - Muscle tenderness
  - Neck pain and tenderness
  - Abnormal electromyography (EMG)
  - Exteroceptive suppression (inhibition of voluntary temporalis muscle EMG activity induced by trigeminal stimulation); this may also be reduced perimenstrually in patients with TTH
  - An increased incidence of MRI white matter lesions
  - Decreased CSF β-endorphin (when severe and chronic).

Table 7.2 Features alerting to a diagnosis of migraine

- A predisposing family history of migraine or prior personal history of travel sickness (e.g. with reading or sitting in the back of vehicles).
- Clear triggering of headache by menstrual cycle, alcohol, insufficient or excessive sleep, and missed meals.
- Premonitory features before the attack (e.g. acute fatigue, excessive yawning, irritability, food cravings, neck ache, etc.)
- Aura, including intermittent sensory symptoms such as numbness or tingling
- Autonomic symptoms such as conjunctival injection, tearing, facial swelling or flushing
- Prominent fatigue or cognitive disturbance during the attack
- Dizziness, e.g. lightheadedness and depersonalization with a sense of feeling 'spaced out', true vertigo during a headache, or visual vertigo where subjects experience dizziness or imbalance when subjected to visual stimuli such as stripes or patterns, road markings, escalators, stairs, converging supermarket aisles, etc.
- Photophobia, phonophobia
- Osmophobia (sensitivity to, or triggering by, smells such as perfumes, cooking, aerosol sprays)
- Worsening of headache with routine physical exercise (e.g. walking up stairs, etc.)

Pathophysiology

- Underlying mechanisms are not understood
- May run in families but is not clearly associated with any specific genotype.
- Previously considered to be due to sustained muscle contraction or secondary to emotion or mental stress, but now considered unlikely.
- Current consensus is peripheral pain mechanisms playing some role in infrequent and frequent TTH, with central pain mechanisms including central sensitization being more important in chronic TTH.
- It is not clear whether episodic and chronic TTH are part of the same disorder or separate entities. Amitriptyline is only effective for chronic and not episodic TTH.

Treatment

- Once a diagnosis of TTH has been established and other more sinister causes of headache excluded, reassurance is all that may be required.
- Treatment trials are limited by diagnostic difficulties.

Pharmacological treatment

- Episodic TTH
  - Simple analgesics usually suffice. These include paracetamol and NSAIDS.
  - Stronger opioid analgesics are not recommended.
  - If the headaches escalate in frequency, it is advisable to change from acute attack to preventative strategies.
- Frequent or chronic TTH
  - Be alert for medication overuse headache
  - Eliminate concurrent medication prior to starting a preventative drug.
  - As a general rule, preventative drugs should be introduced and increased slowly over a number of weeks to minimize adverse effects (see Table 7.3)

Non-pharmacological therapies

In general the evidence base is poor.
- There is limited evidence that cognitive-behavioural therapy (CBT) may help patients who are also facing stress, especially where previous response with pharmacological treatment has been poor.
- Regular exercise may be helpful.
- The evidence for physical therapy including oromandibular treatment is poor.
- There is little evidence to recommend other therapies such as acupuncture, EMG biofeedback, chiropractic, osteopathy or physiotherapy

Table 7.3 Drugs used in frequent or chronic TTH

- Amitriptyline is the treatment of choice for prevention.
- Other TCAs such as dosulepin and nortriptyline may have better side effect profiles.
- Mirtazapine, a noradrenergic and specific serotonergic receptor antagonist, has been shown to be effective. Although less well studied than amitriptyline, it is probably of similar efficacy and possibly better tolerated.
- SSRIs have not been shown to be of any benefit in chronic TTH.
- Topiramate may be of benefit.
- β-Blockers have no role in TTH.
- Avoid the temptation to treat muscle spasm with muscle relaxants (e.g. baclofen, tizanidine, dantrolene) as this does not lead to any clear benefit, and adverse effects are common.
- Avoid benzodiazepines such as diazepam given their ability to cause drug dependence.
- Botulinum toxin has not been shown to help patients with chronic TTH.

Cluster headache and other trigeminal autonomic cephalalgias

Introduction

The trigeminal autonomic cephalalgias (TACs) are a group of primary headache disorders characterized by unilateral head pain that occurs in association with ipsilateral cranial autonomic features. They include cluster headache (CH), paroxysmal hemicrania (PH) and short-lasting unilateral neuralgiform headache attacks with conjunctival injection and tearing (SUNCT). The TACs differ in attack duration and frequency as well as the response to therapy (Table 8.1). The importance of recognizing these syndromes resides in their excellent but highly selective response to treatment.

Cluster headache

CH is a strictly unilateral headache that occurs in association with cranial autonomic features. It is an excruciating syndrome and is probably one of the most painful conditions known, with female patients describing each attack as being worse than childbirth. In most patients, it has a striking circannual and circadian periodicity.

Epidemiology
- The prevalence of CH is estimated to be 0.2%.
- The male: female ratio is 2.5–7.2:1.
- It can begin at any age, though the most common age of onset is the 3rd or 4th decade of life.

Clinical features
Several of the terms relating to CH can be confusing and require defining:
- A *cluster headache or attack* is an individual episode of pain that can last from a few minutes to some hours.
- A *cluster bout or period* refers to the duration over which recurrent cluster attacks are occurring; it usually lasts some weeks or months.
- A *remission* is the pain-free period between two cluster bouts.

CH is a disorder with highly distinctive clinical features. These features are dealt with under 2 major headings: the cluster attack and the cluster bout.

The cluster attack
- The attacks have an abrupt onset and cessation. They are strictly unilateral, though they may alternate sides.
- The pain is excruciatingly severe. It is located mainly around the orbital and temporal regions, though any part of the head can be affected.
- The headache usually lasts 45–90min, but can range from 15min to 3h.

Table 8.1 Clinical features of the trigeminal autonomic cephalalgias

	Cluster headache	Paroxysmal hemicrania	SUNCT
Sex F:M	1:2.5–7.2	1.6–2.4:1	1:1.5
Pain:			
Type	Stabbing, boring	Throbbing, boring, stabbing	Burning, stabbing, sharp
Severity	Excruciating	Excruciating	Severe to excruciating
Site	Orbit, temple	Orbit, temple	Periorbital
Attack frequency	1/alternate day–/day	1–40/day (>5/day for more than half the time)	3–200/day
Duration of attack	15–180min	2–30min	5–240s
Autonomic features	Yes	Yes	Yes[†]
Migrainous features*	Yes	Yes	Very rarely
Alcohol trigger	Yes	Occasional	No
Cutaneous triggers	No	No	Yes
Indometacin effect	–	++	–
Abortive treatment	Sumatriptan injection Sumatriptan or zolmitriptan nasal spray Oxygen	Nil	Nil
Prophylactic treatment	Verapamil Methysergide Lithium Corticosteroids	Indomethacin	Lamotrigine Topiramate Gabapentin IV lidocaine

*Nausea, photophobia or phonophobia.

++Absolute response to indomethacin.

[†]Prominent conjunctival injection **and** lacrimation by definition.

SUNCT = short-lasting unilateral neuralgiform headache attacks with conjunctival injection and tearing.

- The signature feature of CH is the association with cranial autonomic symptoms (see Table 8.2). The autonomic features are transient, lasting only for the duration of the attack, with the exception of partial Horner's syndrome; ptosis or miosis may rarely persist, especially after frequent attacks.
- Migrainous symptoms, such as nausea, photophobia and phonophobia, may be seen, as can aura.
- In contrast to migraine, patients are very often agitated or restless, or even aggressive in attacks.
- The cluster attack frequency varies between one every alternate day to three daily, although some have up to eight daily.
- The condition can have a striking circadian rhythmicity, with some patients reporting that the attacks occur at the same time each day.
- Alcohol, glyceryl trinitrate, exercise, elevated environmental temperature and the smell of volatile agents are recognized precipitants of acute cluster attacks.
- Alcohol induces acute attacks, usually within an hour of intake, in the vast majority of sufferers, contrasting with migraine sufferers who generally have headache some hours after alcohol intake. Alcohol triggers attacks during a cluster bout, but not in a remission.
- Allergies, food sensitivities, reproductive hormonal changes and stress do not appear to have any significant role in precipitating attacks.

The cluster bout or period

- CH is classified according to the duration of the bout:
  - About 80–90% of patients have e*pisodic cluster headache* (ECH), which is diagnosed when they experience recurrent bouts, each with a duration of more than a week, separated by remissions lasting >1 month.
  - 10–20% of patients have *chronic cluster headache* (CCH) in which either no remission occurs within 1 year or the remissions last <1 month.
- Most patients with ECH have one or two annual cluster periods, each lasting between 1 and 3 months.
- Often, a striking circannual periodicity is seen with the cluster periods, with the bouts occurring in the same month of the year.

Table 8.2 The International Classification of Headache Disorders II (ICHD-II) diagnostic criteria for cluster headache

Diagnostic criteria

A. At least 5 attacks fulfilling B–D.

B. Severe or very severe unilateral orbital, supraorbital and/or temporal pain lasting 15–180min if untreated.

C. Headache is accompanied by at least one of the following:
1. ipsilateral conjunctival injection and/or lacrimation
2. ipsilateral nasal congestion and/or rhinorrhoea
3. forehead and facial sweating
4. ipsilateral eyelid oedema
5. ipsilateral forehead and facial sweating
6. ipsilateral miosis and/or ptosis
7. a sense of restlessness or agitation

D. Attacks have a frequency from 1 every other day to 8 per day.

E. Not attributed to another disorder

Episodic cluster headache

Description:

Occurs in periods lasting 7 days to 1 year separated by pain-free periods lasting ≥1 month

Diagnostic criteria:

All fulfilling criteria A–E above
At least 2 cluster periods lasting from 7 to 365 days and separated by pain-free remissions of ≥ 1 month.

Chronic cluster headache

Description:

Attacks occur for >1 year without remission or with remissions lasting <1 month.

Diagnostic criteria:

All fulfilling criteria A–E above
Attacks recur over >1 year without remission periods or with remission periods <1 month

Natural history

- Although there is a paucity of literature on the long-term prognosis of CH, the available evidence suggests that it is a lifelong disorder in the majority of patients.
- About 1/10 of patients with ECH evolved into CCH whereas 1/3 of patients with CCH transformed into ECH.
- A substantial proportion of patients develop longer remission periods as they age.

Differential diagnosis

- The main differential diagnoses to consider are: secondary causes of CH, other TACs and migraine (see Table 8.3)
- Symptomatic CH has been described with infectious, vascular and neoplastic intracranial lesions. Any atypical features in the history or abnormalities on neurological examination (with the exception of partial Horner's syndrome) warrant further investigations to search for organic causes.
- Differentiating between migraine and CH can be difficult in some cases as unilaterality of pain and presence of migrainous and autonomic symptoms are features common to both. The features that can be useful in distinguishing CH from migraine include:
  - relatively short duration of headache
  - rapid onset and cessation
  - circadian periodicity
  - precipitation within an hour, rather than several hours, by alcohol
  - restlessness or agitation during the attack
  - clustering of attacks with intervening remissions in ECH.

Investigations

- The diagnosis of CH is made entirely on the basis of a good clinical history and a detailed neurological examination.
- It can be very difficult to dissect clinically the secondary causes from primary CH, and therefore an MRI scan of the brain is a reasonable screening investigation.
- Consider a trial of indometacin to exclude PH (see section on Paroxysmal hemicrania)

Table 8.3 Differential diagnoses of cluster headache

- Primary headache syndromes:
    - Migraine
    - Paroxysmal hemicrania
    - SUNCT syndrome
    - Hemicrania continua
    - Hypnic headache
- Secondary causes of cluster headache
    - Vascular abnormalities
    - Tumours (particularly pituitary)
    - Infection
    - Traumatic or surgery
- Secondary headache syndromes
    - Tolosa–Hunt syndrome
    - Temporal arteritis
    - Raeder's paratrigeminal neuralgia

Management

General measures and patient education

- Abstain from taking alcohol during the cluster bout.
- Avoid prolonged exposure to volatile substances, such as solvents and oil-based paints.
- Avoid afternoon naps as sleep can precipitate attacks in some patients.

Abortive agents

Because the pain of CH builds up so rapidly, the most efficacious agents are those that involve parentral or pulmonary administration (Table 8.4.)

Triptans:

- SC sumatriptan 6mg is the drug of choice. It has a rapid effect and high response rate. In CH, unlike in migraine, SC sumatriptan can be prescribed at a frequency of bd, on a long-term basis if necessary, without risk of tachyphylaxis or rebound.
- Sumatriptan 20mg nasal spray and zolmitriptan 5mg nasal spray are both more effective than placebo, though they are less likely to work than the injection.
- Oral triptans are generally ineffective, and regular use may induce medication overuse headache in susceptible patients, so that this approach is generally not recommended.

Oxygen:

- Inhalation of 100% oxygen, at 7–12l/min, is rapidly effective in relieving pain in the majority of sufferers. It should be inhaled continuously for 15–20min via a non-rebreathing facial mask.

Octreotide:

- SC octreotide 100mcg is moderately effective in the treatment of acute CH attacks and may have a particular utility in patients who are unresponsive to or intolerant of triptans and oxygen.

Lidocaine:

- Lidocaine solution 20–60mg, given as nasal drops (4–6% lidocaine solution) or a spray deep in the nostril on the painful side, results in mild to moderate relief in most patients, though only a few patients obtain complete pain relief.

Other drugs:

- Oral or rectal ergotamine is generally too slow in onset to provide meaningful relief in a timely manner.
- Opiates, NSAIDs and combination analgesics have no role in the acute management of CH.

Table 8.4 Abortive management of cluster headache

Good efficacy	• Sumatriptan SC injection 6mg (max twice daily for the duration of the cluster bout) • Oxygen 100% at 7–12l/min for 15–30min
Moderate efficacy	• Sumatriptan nasal spray 20mg or zolmitriptan nasal spray 5mg (max thrice daily for the duration of the cluster bout) • Octreotide SC injection 100mcg
Poor efficacy or unproven	• Ergotamine tablets or suppository • Intranasal lidocaine

Preventive treatments

The aim of preventive therapy is to produce a rapid suppression of attacks and to maintain that remission with minimal side effects until the cluster bout is over, or for a longer period in patients with chronic cluster headache (Table 8.5).

Short-term prevention

Patients with either short bouts, perhaps in weeks, or in whom one wishes to control the attack frequency quickly, can benefit from short-term prevention. These medicines are distinguished by the fact that they cannot be used in the long term and thus may require replacement by long-term agents in many patients.

Corticosteroids

- Corticosteroids are highly efficacious and the most rapid-acting of the preventative agents.
- Treatment should be limited to a short intensive course of 2–3 weeks in tapering doses because of the potential for side effects.
- Patients are started on oral prednisolone 1mg/kg to a maximum of 60mg once daily for 5 days, and thereafter the dose decreased by 10mg every 3 days.
- Unfortunately, relapse almost invariably occurs as the dose is tapered. For this reason, corticosteroids are used as an initial therapy in conjunction with preventives, until the latter are effective.

Methysergide

- Methysergide is a potent prophylactic agent for the treatment of CH.
- It is an ideal choice in patients with short cluster bouts that last <4–5 months.
- Doses up to 12mg daily can be used if tolerated (hospital supervision only). Patients are started on 1mg od and the daily dose then increased by 1mg every 3 days (in a tds regime) until the daily dose is 5mg; thereafter, the dose is incremented by 1mg every 5 days.
- Prolonged treatment has been associated with rare fibrotic reactions (retroperitoneal, pulmonary, pleural and cardiac). If prolonged therapy is required, a drug holiday of 1month after every 6 months is necessary, and the patient needs to be checked for evidence of pulmonary, cardiac, renal or abdominal pathology annually.

Greater occipital nerve (GON) injection

- Injection of local anaesthetic and corticosteroid around the GON on the affected side can abort a bout of cluster headache. This is an excellent short-term strategy, with only very modest, infrequent side effects.

Table 8.5 Preventive management of cluster headache

Short-term prevention (for ECH)	Long-term prevention (for prolonged bouts of ECH or CCCH)
Prednisolone (transitional only)	Verapamil
Methysergide	Lithium
Daily (nocturnal) ergotamine[†]	Methysergide
Verapamil	Valproate*
Greater occipital nerve injection	Topiramate[§]
Valproate*	Gabapentin[§]
Melatonin*	Melatonin*
Topiramate[§]	

*Limited or negative data.
[†]Patients with predictable nocturnal headaches only.
[§]Unproven but promising.

Long-term prevention

Verapamil

- Verapamil is the preventive drug of choice in both ECH and CCH.
- Clinical experience has demonstrated that higher doses than those used in cardiological indications are needed. Dosages commonly employed range from 240 to 960mg daily in divided doses.
- Verapamil can cause heart block by slowing conduction in the atrio-ventricular node. Observing for PR interval prolongation on ECG can monitor potential development of heart block.
- After performing a baseline ECG, patients are usually started on 80mg tds and thereafter the total daily dose is increased in increments of 80mg every 10–14 days. An ECG is performed prior to each increment. The dose is increased until the cluster attacks are suppressed, side effects intervene or the maximum dose of 960mg daily is achieved.
- About 20% of CH patients on verapamil have cardiac conduction problems, and these can develop after months of stable dosing and are not dose dependent. Thus, an ECG needs to be performed every 6 months with long-term therapy.

Lithium

- Lithium is an effective agent for CH prophylaxis, though the response is less robust in ECH than in CCH.
- Renal and thyroid function tests are performed prior to initiation of therapy. Patients are then started on 300mg twice daily and the dose titrated, aiming for a serum lithium level in the upper part of the therapeutic range. Most patients will benefit from dosages of 600–1200mg daily.
- The concomitant use of NSAIDs, diuretics and carbamazepine is contraindicated.

Other drugs

- Though topiramate, sodium valproate, pizotifen and gabapentin are often used, they are of as yet unproven efficacy.

Surgery

- This is a last-resort measure in treatment-resistant patients.
- Procedures may be destructive, such as pterygopalatine ganglion or trigeminal ganglion procedures, or even trigeminal nerve root section.
- Most recentlym neurostimulation therapies with either deep-brain stimulation of the posterior hypothalamic region or ONS have emerged. These approaches are very promising and especially ONS offers a more acceptable side effect profile than destructive and invasive approaches.

Table 8.6 Pathophysiology of trigeminal autonomic cephalalgias

- Any pathophysiological construct for TACs must account for the three major clinical features characteristic of the conditions that comprise this group:
  - Trigeminal distribution pain.
  - Ipsilateral autonomic features.
  - The curious periodicity or regularity that often marks the attack incidence.
- The pain-producing innervation of the cranium projects through branches of the trigeminal and upper cervical nerves to the trigeminocervical complex, from whence nociceptive pathways project to higher centres. This implies an integral role for the ipsilateral trigeminal nociceptive pathways in TACs.
- The ipsilateral autonomic features suggest cranial parasympathetic activation (lacrimation, rhinorrhoea, nasal congestion and eyelid oedema) and sympathetic hypofunction (ptosis and miosis).
- It has been suggested that the pathophysiology of the TACs revolves around the trigeminal autonomic reflex.
  - There is considerable experimental animal literature to document that stimulation of trigeminal afferents can result in cranial autonomic outflow, the trigeminal autonomic reflex.
  - Some degree of cranial autonomic symptomatology is a normal physiologic response to cranial nociceptive input, and patients with other headache syndromes often report these symptoms.
  - The distinction between the TACs and other headache syndromes is the degree of cranial autonomic activation, not its presence.
- The cranial autonomic symptoms may be prominent in the TACs due to a central disinhibition of the trigeminal autonomic reflex.
- Supporting evidence has emerged from functional imaging studies: positron emission tomography (PET) studies in CH and PH, and functional MRI studies in SUNCT syndrome have demonstrated hypothalamic activation.
  - Importantly, the involvement of posterior hypothalamic structures may account for the rhythmicity or periodicity that is such a hallmark of these conditions.
  - Hypothalamic activation is not seen in episodic and chronic migraine or experimental trigeminal distribution head pain.
  - There are direct hypothalamic–trigeminal connections. There is abundant evidence for a role for the hypothalamus in mediating antinociceptive and autonomic responses.
  - Hence, the TACs are probably due to an abnormality in the hypothalamus with subsequent trigeminovascular and cranial autonomic activation.

Paroxysmal hemicrania

PH is a rare syndrome that responds in a dramatic and absolute fashion to indometacin, thereby underlining the importance of distinguishing it from CH and SUNCT, which are not responsive to indometacin.

Epidemiology

- The prevalence of PH is not known, but the relationship compared with CH is reported to be ~1–3% (1 per 25 000).
- PH predominates in females by a sex ratio of 1.6–2.4:1
- It can begin at any age, though the most common age of onset is the 2nd or 3rd decade of life

Clinical features

- Highly characteristic unilateral, relatively brief, severe attacks of pain associated with cranial autonomic features that recur several times per day.
- The attacks have an abrupt onset and cessation. The pain is strictly unilateral and centred around the orbital and temporal regions, though any part of the head can be affected. It is excruciatingly severe. The headache usually lasts 2–30min. Interictal discomfort or pain is present in up to 60% of patients.
- Attacks of PH invariably occur in association with ipsilateral cranial autonomic features (see Table 8.7).
- Up to 85% of patients report at least one migrainous feature of photophobia, nausea or vomiting during an attack.
- Similar to CH, patients are often restless or agitated during an attack.
- The frequency of attacks in PH is high, ranging from 1-40 daily.
- The attacks occur regularly throughout the 24h period without a preponderance of nocturnal attacks as in CH.
- While the majority of attacks are spontaneous, ~10% of attacks may be precipitated mechanically, either by bending or by rotating the head. Attacks may also be provoked by external pressure against the transverse processes of C4–5, C2 root or the greater occipital nerve. Alcohol ingestion triggers headaches in only 7% of patients
- PH is classified depending on the presence of a remission period:
  - About 20% of patients have *episodic paroxysmal hemicrania* (EPH), which is diagnosed when they experience recurrent bouts, each with a duration of more than a week and separated by remissions lasting ≥1 month.
  - The remaining 80% of patients have *chronic paroxysmal hemicrania* (CPH), in which either no remission occurs within 1 year or the remissions last <1 month.
- Notably, in PH the chronic form dominates the clinical presentation, in contrast to CH in which the episodic form prevails.

Table 8.7 The International Classification of Headache Disorders II (ICHD-II) diagnostic criteria for paroxysmal hemicrania

Diagnostic criteria:

A. PAt least 20 attacks fulfilling B–D.

B. Severe unilateral orbital, supraorbital, or temporal pain lasting 2–30min.

C. Headache is accompanied by at least one of the following:

1. ipsilateral conjunctival injection and/or lacrimation
2. ipsilateral nasal congestion and/or rhinorrhoea
3. forehead and facial sweating
4. ipsilateral eyelid oedema
5. ipsilateral forehead and facial sweating
6. ipsilateral miosis and/or ptosis

D. Attacks have a frequency above 5 per day for more than half the time, although periods with lower frequency may occur

E. Attacks are prevented completely by therapeutic doses of indometacin*

F. Not attributed to another disorder

Episodic paroxysmal headache
Description:
Occurs in periods lasting 7 days to 1 year separated by pain-free periods lasting ≥1 month

Chronic paroxysmal headache
Description:
Attacks occur for >1 year without remission or with remissions lasting <1 month.

*To rule out an incomplete response, indometacin should be used in a dose of ≥150mg daily orally or rectally, or ≥100mg by injection. Smaller doses are often sufficient for maintenance.

Differential diagnosis

- The differential diagnosis includes: symptomatic causes of PH, other TACs and hemicrania continua (HC).
- Symptomatic PH is relatively common and can be caused by diverse pathological processes at various intracranial sites.
- There is a considerable overlap in the clinical phenotype of PH and CH. Though PH differs from CH in not having a male dominance, and having shorter duration of attacks that are more frequent, the utility of these characteristics is limited by the considerable overlap in the two syndromes. In view of this, in all patients diagnosed with TACs a trial of indometacin should be considered at the start of treatment to detect the indometacin-sensitive group
- As 2/3 of PH patients report interictal pain, HC needs to be considered in the differential diagnosis of these cases. HC is a strictly unilateral, continuous headache that is exquisitely responsive to indomethacin.

Investigations

- The diagnosis of PH is made entirely on the basis of a good clinical history and a detailed neurological examination.
- As a relatively high number of symptomatic cases have been reported, an MRI brain scan should be routinely performed in all PH patients.
- The therapeutic trial of oral indometacin is initiated at 25mg tds; if there is no or a partial response after 3 days, the dose is increased to 50mg tds for 10 days; if the index of suspicion is high, then the dose is further increased to 75mg tds for 10 days. Complete resolution of the headache is prompt, usually occurring within 1–2 days of initiating the effective dose, though some patients can take 10 days.
- Injectable indometacin 100mg IM ('indotest') has been proposed as a diagnostic test for PH. The indotest has the advantage that the diagnosis can be rapidly established though it needs further validation at this stage, with placebo-controlled trials in PH and the other TACs.

Management

The treatment of PH is entirely preventive, as attacks are too short and intense for any acute oral treatment to be effective. Indomethacin is the treatment of choice.

Indometacin

- Complete resolution of the headache is prompt, usually occurring within 1–2 days of initiating the effective dose.
- The typical maintenance dose ranges from 25 to 100mg daily, but may vary inter- and intraindividually between 12.5 and 300mg daily, depending on the fluctuation in attack severity. Hence, dosage adjustments may be necessary to address the clinical fluctuations seen in PH.

Table 8.8 Treatment options in paroxysmal hemicrania

• Drug treatments	• Indometacin
	• Other NSAIDs
	• aspirin
	• ibuprofen
	• diclofenac
	• ketoprofen
	• piroxicam β-cyclodextrin
	• Cyclooxygenase-2 inhibitors
	• rofecoxib
	• celecoxib
	• Topiramate
• Surgery	• Local blockades (including GON block)
	• ONS

- On discontinuation, symptoms usually appear within 12h to 2 weeks though during active headache cycles; skipping or even delaying doses may result in the prompt reoccurrence of the headache.
- In patients with EPH, indometacin should be given for slightly longer than the typical headache bout and then gradually tapered.
- In patients with CPH, long-term treatment is usually necessary; however, long-lasting remissions have been reported in rare patients following cessation of indometacin. Hence drug withdrawal should be advised at least once every 6 months.
- The most common serious side effect of indometacin is the development of peptic ulcers. Gastrointestinal side effects secondary to indometacin may be treated with antacids, misoprostol, histamine H_2 receptor antagonists or proton pump inhibitors, and should always be considered for patients who require long-term treatment.
- Patients who need escalating doses of indometacin to suppress the symptoms, become refractory to treatment with indometacin or require a continuous, high dosage of indometacin may have underlying pathology and need careful diagnostic evaluation for symptomatic causes.
- For patients who cannot tolerate indometacin, one faces a difficult challenge. No other drug is consistently effective in PH. Some response is seen with a range of other NSAIDs; however, this is usually not helpful. Other drug therapies that have been reported to be effective in PH are reviewed in Table 8.8.

Natural history and prognosis

- Though there is a paucity of literature on the natural history of PH, the available evidence suggests that it is a lifelong condition
- Patients can expect sustained efficacy of indometacin treatment without developing tachyphylaxis, though about 1/4 develop gastrointestinal side effects.
- Indometacin does not seem to alter the condition in the long term, though a significant proportion of patients can decrease the dose of indometacin required to maintain a pain-free state.

SUNCT

Short-lasting unilateral neuralgiform headache attacks with conjunctival injection and tearing (SUNCT), as its name implies, is a disorder characterized by strictly unilateral, severe, neuralgic attacks centred on the ophthalmic trigeminal distribution that are brief in duration and occur in association with conjunctival injection and lacrimation.

Epidemiology

- The prevalence and incidence of SUNCT are not known, though it is a very rare syndrome,
- SUNCT has a slight male predominance, with a sex ratio of 1.5:1,
- The typical age of onset is between 35 and 65 years, with a mean of 48 years and a range between 10 and 77 years,

Clinical features

- The attacks are strictly unilateral, though may alternate sides.
- The pain is usually maximal in the ophthalmic distribution of the trigeminal nerve, but can radiate to any part of the head. It has an excruciating intensity and a neuralgic or throbbing quality.
- The individual attacks are relatively brief, lasting between 5 and 240s.
- Three different types of pain have been described (see Table 8.10)
- By definition, all SUNCT patients had both ipsilateral conjunctival injection and lacrimation associated with their attacks (see Table 8.9).
- Migrainous features are not usually associated with SUNCT
- The attack frequency during the symptomatic phase varies immensely between sufferers and within an individual sufferer. Attacks may be as infrequent as once a day or less, to >60/h.
- The majority of patients can precipitate attacks by touching certain trigger zones within the trigeminal innervated distribution and, occasionally, even from an extra-trigeminal territory. Precipitants include touching the face or scalp, washing, shaving, eating, chewing, brushing teeth, talking and coughing. Unlike in trigeminal neuralgia, most patients have no refractory period.

Table 8.9 The International Classification of Headache Disorders II (ICHD-II) diagnostic criteria for short-lasting unilateral neuralgiform headache attacks with conjunctival injection and tearing (SUNCT)

A. At least 20 attacks fulfilling criteria B–E

B. Attacks of unilateral orbital, supraorbital or temporal stabbing or pulsating pain lasting 5–240s

C. Pain is accompanied by ipsilateral conjunctival injection and lacrimation

D. Attacks occur with a frequency from 3–200/day

E. Not attributed to another disorder

Table 8.10 Types of SUNCT syndrome

- Single stabs
- Groups of stabs
- Saw-tooth pattern in which repetitive spike-like paroxysms occur without reaching the pain-free baseline between the individual spikes

Differential diagnosis

- The differential diagnosis of very brief headaches includes: SUNCT (primary and secondary forms); trigeminal neuralgia; primary stabbing headache; and PH.
- Secondary SUNCT is typically seen with either posterior fossa or pituitary gland lesions. In symptomatic SUNCT secondary to pituitary tumours, the headache symptoms can precede the pituitary symptoms by 3–10 years.
- Differentiating SUNCT from trigeminal neuralgia can be challenging in some cases, as there is a considerable overlap in the clinical phenotypes of the two syndromes. Table 8.11 outlines the useful differentiating features.
- Primary stabbing headache refers to brief, sharp or jabbing pains in the head that occur either as a single episode or in brief repeated volleys. The pain usually lasts a fraction of a second but can persist for up to 1min. These headaches are generally easily distinguishable from SUNCT:
  - In primary stabbing headache there is a female preponderance.
  - The site and radiation of pain often vary between attacks.
  - The majority of the attacks tend to be spontaneous.
  - Cranial autonomic features are absent.
  - The attacks commonly subside with the administration of indometacin.
- PH does not exhibit cutaneous triggering and is responsive to indometacin, unlike SUNCT.

Investigations

- The association of secondary SUNCT with pituitary and posterior fossa abnormalities emphasizes the absolute need for a cranial MRI, including an adequate view of the pituitary.
- These patients should also have a screen for basal pituitary hormone profile.
- Perform a therapeutic trial of indomethacin to exclude an indometacin-responsive headache.

Natural history and prognosis

- The natural history of SUNCT is poorly understood.
- It appears to be a lifelong disorder once it starts, though more prospective data are needed.
- The syndrome itself is not fatal and does not cause any long-term neurological sequelae.

Table 8.11 Differentiating features of SUNCT and trigeminal neuralgia

Feature	SUNCT	Trigeminal neuralgia
Gender ratio (M:F)	1.5:1	1:2
Site of pain	V_1	$V_{2/3}$
Duration (seconds)	5–240	<5
Autonomic features	Prominent	Sparse or none
Refractory period	Absent	Present
Response to carbamazepine	Partial	Complete
Evidence of vascular loop on MRI	7%	47–90%

Table 8.12 Management of SUNCT

Drug treatments	• Long-term prevention
	• Lamotrigine
	• Topiramate
	• Gabapentin
	• Carbamazepine
	• Short-term prevention
	• IV lidocaine
Surgery	• Local blocks (including GON block)
	• Hypothalamic stimulation (experimental)

Cervicogenic headache

Introduction

Cervicogenic headache (CGH) is a headache originating from a source in the neck. First described in 1913, there remains controversy and confusion on all matters pertaining to the topic. Although in the minority, some neurologists promote CGH as a major cause of headache. It should be considered in chronic unilateral headache, without side shift, where pain starts in the neck or occipital region and is associated with tenderness of cervical paraspinal tissues ipsilateral to the headache and where no other diagnosis seems likely.

Epidemiology

- Prevalence estimates range from 0.4 to 2.5% of the general population
- 15–20% of patients with chronic headaches have CGH.
- Mean age is 43 years, with a 4:1 female disposition.

Clinical features

- Almost all pathology affecting the cervical spine had been implicated, but no specific imaging features have correlated with CGH.
- The pain may be felt almost anywhere on the head or face, but behind the eye is quite typical.
- Patients may feel the problem is in the eye, ear, sinuses or teeth, depending on where the pain is referred, and seek out specialist advice from appropriate specialists who may not be familiar with CGH.
- Practical diagnostic criteria are not available.
  - In 1983 Sjaastad introduced the term 'cervicogenic headache' and in 1990 published diagnostic criteria.
  - The IHS classification of CGH is shown in Table 9.1.
  - The IHS criteria attempt a strict and scientific definition of this disorder and fail to encompass what is a subtle and subjective clinical entity.
  - The lack of ready availability of diagnostic nerve blocks makes these criteria unhelpful for general clinic practice. Basing a diagnosis on the response to a treatment, a nerve block, is potentially misleading.

Differential diagnosis

- HC
- Primary stabbing headache
- SUNCT. Neck disorders may trigger an attack
- CPH. Neck disorders may trigger an attack
- CH
- Migraine
- Occipital neuralgia (IHS diagnostic criteria exist but a controversial entity)
- Tension headache (rarely)

Table 9.1 IHS diagnosis of cervicogenic headache

A. Pain, referred from a source in the neck and perceived in one or more regions of the head and/or face, fulfilling criteria C and D.

B. Clinical, laboratory and/or imaging evidence of a disorder or lesion within the cervical spine or soft tissues of the neck known to be, or generally accepted as, a valid cause of headache.

C. Evidence that the pain can be attributed to the neck disorder or lesion based on at least one of the following:
  1. Demonstration of physical signs that implicate a source in the neck
  2. Abolition of headache following diagnostic blockade of a cervical structure or its nerve supply using placebo or other adequate controls.

D. Pain resolves within 3 months after successful treatment of the causative disorder or lesion.

Notes:

- Tumours, fractures, infections and rheumatoid arthritis of the upper cervical spine have not been validated formally as a cause of headache, but are nevertheless accepted as valid causes when demonstrated to be so in individual cases.

- Cervical spondylosis and osteochondritis are NOT accepted as valid causes fulfilling criterion B. When myofascial tender spots are the cause, the headache should be coded under 2. Tension-type headache.

- Clinical signs acceptable for criterion C1 must have demonstrated reliability and validity. The future task is the identification of such reliable and valid operational tests.

- Clinical features such as neck pain, focal neck tenderness, history of neck trauma, mechanical exacerbation of pain, unilaterality, co-existing shoulder pain, reduced range of motion in the neck, nuchal onset, nausea, vomiting, photophobia, etc. are not unique to CGH. These may be features of CGH but they do not define the relationship between the disorder and the source of the headache.

- Abolition of headache means complete relief of headache, indicating a score of zero on a visual analogue scale (VAS). Nevertheless, acceptable as fulfilling criterion C2 is ≥90% reduction in pain to a level of <5 on a 100-point VAS.

- Major symptoms and signs (points 1 and 2 are obligatory. In point 2 at least one of criteria A–C is required).

Pathogenesis

- The sensory supply to the face and the scalp back to the vertex is through the trigeminal nerve.
- The occipital region and neck are supplied by C2 and C3 (Fig. 9.1).
- C1 is mostly absent or rudimentary.
- Cervical and trigeminal sensory inputs overlap in the trigemino-cervical complex. Pain can be referred from one area to another.
  - Spinal levels at C2/C3 may influence the genesis of headache pain posteriorly via the occipital nerve.
  - Spinal levels at C2/C3 may influence the genesis of headache pain anteriorly via the cervico-trigeminal pathway.
  - This overlap does not apply to the lower cervical roots and so conditions affecting the lower neck do not produce headache.
  - Cervical–trigeminal interactions may aggravate an already established pattern of primary headache.
  - Trigeminal nociception can facilitate cervical perception and so any 'abnormality' found in the neck ipsilateral to a cranial source of headache might be secondary to the headache.

Treatment

- Various therapies have been used, but in general CGH is unresponsive to common headache medication.
- Small non-controlled cases series have reported moderate success with surgery and injections.
- A few RCTs and a number of case series support:
  - Cervical manipulation:
  - Transcutaneous electrical nerve stimulation
  - Botulinum toxin injection
  - Steroid injection.

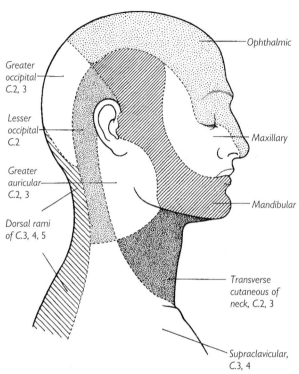

Fig. 9.1 Cutaneous sensory supply of the head and neck.
Reproduced from *Gray's Anatomy*, (1973) p. 1009, with permission from Elsevier.

Chapter 10

Headache attributed to head or neck trauma

Introduction

Post-traumatic headache (PTH) is estimated to affect 30–90% of patients with mild head injury (75% of head injuries are mild). Most PTH resolves within 6 months, but 25% persists. Although data are contested, PTH is more prevalent and lasts longer after mild head injury than after more severe head injury.

Establishing a relationship of headache with the trauma

- Arbitrary criteria are set that to be attributable to head injury the headache should start within 7 days (see Table 10.1).
- Since the aetiology of PTH is not understood, a short latency is reasonable within this definition.
- It is very difficult to attribute a headache that develops after weeks or months when most PTHs have patterns similar to migraine or TTH and these headache types are very common.
- Headache after an injury may be an exacerbation of a pre-existing primary headache (such as migraine or TTH) or a new primary headache precipitated by the injury.
  - When an existing primary headache has been made worse by the injury it can either be diagnosed as the primary headache type or also given a second diagnosis of PTH.
  - The latter option is most appropriate if the headache became worse very soon after the injury, if it was made much worse by the injury and if the headache improves after recovery from the injury.
  - More rarely, migraine (with or without aura) can be triggered by mild head injury. Often adolescents after sports-related head injuries, e.g. football and rugby, have multiple migraine with aura attacks triggered only by impact, sometimes termed 'footballer's migraine'. A family history of migraine may be a predisposing factor.
  - Episodes of transient hemiplegia and headache may very rarely be induced by minor head injury. This has mainly been reported in children and adolescents from families with familial hemiplegia. Rare cases of coma and even death from massive cerebral oedema have also been reported.
  - Rarely HC may be triggered by mild head injury.
  - There is only one reported case of post-traumatic cluster headache.

Classification of post-traumatic headache

Acute post-traumatic headache (lasting <3 months post-injury)

- The aetiology is unknown.
- This may follow either mild or moderate/severe head injury, or whiplash injury.
- Most PTH is from mild head injuries and has features of TTH.

Table 10.1 IHS classification of post-traumatic headache

	Acute	**Chronic**
Onset	Within 7 days of injury (or regaining of consciousness)	
Duration	Less than 3 months following head injury	More than 3 months following head injury
Attributed to mild head injury	Loss of consciousness <30min GCS 13–15 Symptoms and/or signs of concussion	
Attributed to moderate/severe head injury	At least one of: Loss of consciousness >30min GCS <13 Post-traumatic amnesia for >48h Imaging demonstrative of a traumatic brain lesion	
Attributed to whiplash injury	History of whiplash associated at the time with neck pain	

Chronic post-traumatic headache (lasting >3 months post-injury)

- May follow mild or moderate/severe head injury or after whiplash, but there is little correlation with the severity of the injury.
- Most (77%) chronic PTH following mild head injury has characteristics of TTH, but migraine-like headache may also develop.
- Can occur without any abnormalities:
  - Neurological examination is normal.
  - Investigations such as neuroimaging, CSF, EEG, evoked potentials, vestibular function tests and neuropsychological testing are normal.
  - There is no evidence that abnormalities in any of the above changes prognosis or directs treatment, so these investigations should not be used routinely once a secondary cause of the headache has been excluded.
- The aetiology is unknown, but suggestions are:
  - Cortical dysfunction altering the neuronal threshold for pain.
  - Dysregulation of brainstem nociceptive pathways.
- The inverse relationship between severity of injury and persistence of symptoms goes against an organic basis. Psychological factors (Table 10.2) associated with longer duration of symptoms may suggest a more functional basis to ongoing symptoms.
- It is usually part of an ongoing post-concussion syndrome.
- Chronic PTH is associated with more disability than other chronic headaches.

Post-traumatic secondary headaches

A secondary cause for PTH should always be excluded. This is more likely after moderate or severe head trauma, but some (e.g. arterial dissection and dural tears) may occur with relatively trivial injuries.

The following should be considered:
- Scalp lacerations/local trauma.
- Subdural haematomas (up to 1% incidence after mild head injury).
- Extradural haematomas (up to 1% incidence after mild head injury).
- Low CSF pressure (volume): trauma can cause CSF leak through a dural tear.
- Carotid or vertebral artery dissection.
- Cerebral venous thrombosis.

Post-concussion syndrome

- More commonly follows minor head injury.
- Comprises one or more symptom and sign (Table 10.3) of which headache is a part.
- 4 weeks after mild head injury 20% complain of difficulty concentrating and 20% complain of poor memory.
- The mechanism is unknown. There probably is a neuropathological substrate, but psychological factors and ongoing litigation may exacerbate symptoms.

Table 10.2 Risk factors for chronic headache after mild head injury

- Female
- Age >40 years
- Lower socio-economic status
- Lower education level
- Pre-injury unemployment
- Prior head injury
- Minor headache injury (no or minimal amnesia, no or minimal loss of consciousness)
- Psychological /psychiatric factors, e.g. post-traumatic depression, pre-morbid personality traits
- Previous history of headache
- There is no good evidence that ongoing litigation and impending settlement is associated with prolongation of chronic PTH or of whiplash symptoms
- Ongoing litigation may sometimes increase stress levels and may contribute to the persistence of symptoms, but often they do not resolve with settlement of litigation
- There are some patients whose symptoms may be exaggerated due to malingering, seeking exaggerated compensation claims, secondary gain and psychosocial factors

Table 10.3 Features of the post-concussion syndrome

Symptom	Frequency
• Headaches	<90%
• Dizziness	<53%
• Blurred vision	14%
• Photophobia	7%
• Phonophobia	15%
• Anosmia	5%

• Psychological and somatic symptoms:
  • Irritability/anxiety/depression
  • Personality change
  • Fatigue
  • Decreased libido
  • Poor sleep
  • Memory loss/poor concentration
	<85%

Headache following whiplash injury

- Sudden and significant acceleration/deceleration movement of the neck from rear-end or side-on motor vehicle accidents (whiplash) often accompanies head trauma and can be associated with headaches.
- Whiplash describes the mechanism of the trauma, not subsequent symptoms. Up to 80% of patients complain of headache following whiplash injury.
- Many also complain of dizziness, upper limb paraesethesia, psychological and cognitive symptoms.
- The aetiology for this without any structural abnormality on imaging is uncertain, but may involve activation of C2 afferents that have central connections with the trigeminal nucleus caudalis which may alter brainstem nociceptive reflexes.
- Persistent headaches should be treated as for other chronic PTH.

Prognosis

- 25% of patients have headache lasting for >6 months.
- There is no direct correlation between severity of head injury and persistence and severity of headache or symptoms of the post-concussion syndrome.
- Higher socio-economic status, employment and higher level of education predict return to work at 3 months, and other factors may predict the persistence of PTH as outlined in Table 10.3.

Investigation of post-traumatic headache

- Exclude secondary causes with appropriate investigations (neuroimaging ± LP) for:
  - all moderate/severe head injury.
  - mild head injury with subsequent acute neurological deterioration.
  - ongoing symptoms after mild head injury suggestive of a secondary cause such as low CSF pressure headache.

Treatment of post-traumatic headache

- There is no RCT evidence to support any one treatment modality.
- Treatment in the acute phase may reduce progression to chronic PTH and its associated disability.
- A multidisciplinary approach is recommended including supportive psychotherapy and encouraging a return to work.
- Treat TTH and migraine with usual symptomatic and preventative medication appropriate for the headache type. Amitriptyline may be a good option, particularly if the patient also has depression.
- Depression and anxiety (as co-morbid features or as part of the post-concussion syndrome) should be actively treated.
- Avoid analgesic overuse:
  - <42% of patients with chronic PTH overuse analgesics which may cause a medication overuse headache.
  - Discontinuation of the analgesics will by itself improve headache in about half of patients, and still more will then respond to conventional prophylactic medication.

Headache due to disorders of CSF pressure

Idiopathic intracranial hypertension

Idiopathic intracranial hypertension ((IIH) or benign intracranial hypertension) is the clinical syndrome of raised intracranial pressure without ventricular enlargement for which no cause can be found. The syndrome of idiopathic intracranial hypertension without papilloedema is recognized, but diagnosis and management are controversial. The term secondary intracranial hypertension should be used for cases with a clear causative factor. The term 'benign' is a misnomer as permanent visual loss occurs in ~10%.

Epidemiology

Incidence: 1–2 per 100 000, rising to ~20 per 100 000 amongst young, overweight women. Female:male ratio ~10:1.

Clinical features

Symptoms

- Headache
  - The most common symptom, affecting >90% of adults with IIH.
  - Rates amongst children seem to be lower.
  - Typically progressive over days or weeks, the pain is often worse in the morning, but classical features of raised intracranial pressure are often absent.
  - Retrobulbar, occipital, temporal and hemicranial as well as generalized locations are described.
  - The pain may be intermittent or constant, and varies widely in severity.
  - May mimic or co-exist with migraine or TTH.
- Visual disturbance
  - Presentation may be highly asymmetric.
  - Transient visual obscurations—shadows, patches, blurring or loss of vision in one or both eyes resolving after a few seconds or minutes—often noticed on changing posture, e.g. standing suddenly from bending.
  - Photopsia ('sparkles')—seeing flashes of light.
  - Horizontal diplopia (VI palsy).
  - Visual loss is less common, central vision is usually spared. Patients may be aware of enlargement of their bind spots.
- Tinnitus
  - Intracranial noises affect up to 60%.
  - Often pulsatile, 'whooshing' or roaring in one or both ears.
  - May be worse on lying down.
- Other symptoms
  - Symptoms of meningeal irritation such as nausea (20%), vomiting and photophobia may occur.

Table 11.1 Diagnostic criteria for idiopathic intracranial hypertension

- Intracranial pressure, as measured in the lateral decubitus position, is raised
- Normal CSF composition
- No evidence of hydrocephalus, mass, structural or vascular lesion
- No metabolic, toxic or hormonal cause of raised intracranial pressure identified
- If symptoms or signs are present, they may only indicate those of generalized intracranial hypertension or papilloedema

Table 11.2 Associations with intracranial hypertension

- Only female sex and obesity have been conclusively associated with IIH.
- High rates in pregnancy and oral contraceptive use reflect the predilection of IIH for women of childbearing age.
- Co-exisiting menstrual dysfunction and polycystic ovary disease are common, but no specific hormone abnormality has been identified.
- A multitude of conditions have been reported in association with the clinical syndrome (see table 11.3), but may occur by chance.

- Rarely patients may complain of neck, back, shoulder or radicular pain.
- Asymptomatic presentation is not uncommon; the patient may be referred via their optician with papilloedema found on routine examination.

Examination

The IIH patient is alert, with a normal neurological examination or:

- Papilloedema—often asymmetrical and may be unilateral.
- Sixth nerve palsy—examine ocular movements for horizontal diplopia
- Enlarged blind spot or visual field defect
- Relative afferent pupillary defect (RAPD)—examine the pupil responses

Visual function assessment

- Best corrected visual acuity.
- Check colour vision—testing with pseudo-isochromatic plates (e.g. Ishihara) is quick and easy but be aware of inherited colour blindness (≤10% males, ≤0.5% females).
- Visual fields—always supplement confrontation testing with formal perimetry: Goldmann or automated (e.g. Humphrey) fields.
  - Abnormalities are common even in the absence of visual symptoms.
  - The most common defects are enlargement of the blind spot, generalized constriction, inferior arcuate defects and nasal 'steps'.
- Contrast sensitivity testing (e.g. Pelli–Robson charts) may reveal minor defects even if acuity is normal, but is not widely used.
- Slit-lamp examination of retina and optic nerve
  - Dilate the pupils and obtain photographs if possible.
  - Look for blurred disc margins, distended retinal veins with absent spontaneous pulsations, haemorrhages and exudates.
  - Optic atrophy may occur in longstanding disease.
  - Congenital anomalous variations of the optic nerve head (e.g. drusen) can be difficult—an expert neuro-ophthalmology opinion is essential.
  - Optic nerve ultrasound or retinal tomography (e.g. laser scanning) may add information but cannot replace thorough assessment of visual function.

Investigations

IIH is a diagnosis of exclusion.

- MRI (or CT) brain imaging.
  - Empty sella and swelling of the optic nerve are common findings in an otherwise normal scan.
  - Venography is mandatory to exclude venous sinus thrombosis, which can present with an identical clinical picture.
  - Narrowing of the transverse sinuses is a common finding and may be difficult to distinguish from thrombus.

Table 11.3 Co-morbid conditions and medications reported in association with IIH

Endocrine
- Corticosteroid treatment and withdrawal
- Levonorgestrel
- Growth hormone
- Tamoxifen
- Danazol
- Anabolic steroids
- Diabetes mellitus
- Thyroid disease
- Hyperparathyroidism
- Polycystic ovary syndrome
- Turner syndrome
- Adrenal insufficiency

Haematological
- Anaemia
- Sickle cell disease
- Prothrombotic states

Antibiotics
- Tetracycline and derivatives
- Nalidixic acid
- Nitrofurantoin
- Penicillin

Vitamin A
- Hyper- and hypovitaminosis A
- Retinoids

NSAIDs
- Indometacin
- Rofecoxib

Other
- Systemic arterial hypertension
- Sleep apnoea
- Systemic lupus erythematosus
- Renal transplant
- Lithium carbonate

- Measurement of CSF pressure
  This is essential for making the diagnosis.
  - LP is safe in the fully conscious patient with no focal neurological deficit and normal brain imaging.
  - Record CSF opening pressure accurately and have more than two manometers handy as pressures are often >40cm.
  - The patient should be as relaxed as possible, ideally with the legs extended.
  - An opening pressure >25cm H_2O is diagnostic. The effect of obesity on CSF pressure is debated. 20–25cm is a grey area.
  - Send CSF for cell count, culture, protein and glucose. A low protein is acceptable.

Pathogenesis

- The cause is unknown.
- Older names such as pseudotumour cerebri and serous meningitis reflect historical attempts to define the pathophysiology.
- Hypotheses have developed around the main determinants of CSF pressure, e.g. excess production, impaired absorption and increased cerebral venous pressure.

Treatment

- The main aim of treatment is to halt or prevent visual loss.
- Lowering the intracranial pressure by direct removal of CSF may provide temporary relief of signs and symptoms, but repeated LPs are no longer used. The CSF is rapidly replaced and the procedure is unpopular with patients.
- Longer term management is controversial. No RCTs have been done. Weight reduction is associated with clinical improvement and should be recommended in all overweight patients

Medical

- Acetazolamide, a carbonic anhydrase inhibitor, has been shown to reduce CSF production and may lower intracranial pressure in IIH.
  - Initial dose is usually 250–500mg daily; can be increased if tolerated.
  - Common side effects are acroparaesthesiae, nausea, altered taste sensation and fatigue. Less common are hypokalaemia, rash and blood count disorders.
  - Other diuretics, e.g. furosemide, are sometimes used.
- Corticosteroids may be effective but are not recommended because of side effects.
- Analgesics are often indicated, but should be used with caution to avoid medication overuse headache.
- Topiramate is sometimes used—also a weak carbonic anhydrase inhibitor and may cause weight loss.

Surgical

- *CSF diversion via shunt* insertion can be sight saving.
  - Practical considerations and neurosurgical expertise determine the choice between ventriculoperitoneal (VP) or lumboperitoneal (LP) shunts.
  - Complications include low-pressure headaches, infections and shunt failure requiring revision.
- *Optic nerve sheath fenestration* has been performed in some centres.
  - A slit made in the dural sheath reduces optic nerve pressure locally and can relieve visual disturbance, but may not treat the other symptoms of IIH.

Table 11.4 A quick guide to IIH managment

Signs and symptoms of raised intracranial hypertension
Neurological exam otherwise normal

↓

Book MRI and MRV
Exclude space-occupying lesion, intracranial disease and venous
sinus thrombosis

↓

Document visual function and perimetry
Refer to neuro-ophthalmology promptly

↓

Perform LP, and record opening and closing CSF pressures
Send CSF for analysis

↓

Check medication, co-morbid conditions
Identify and treat 'secondary' intracranial hypertension

↓

Counsel re weight reduction
Consider acetazolamide and analgesia if symptoms troublesome
Organize regular review even if apparently stable

↓

Act quickly if vision is deteriorating—seek urgent opinion re surgery
'Buy time' with repeat LP if necessary

Table 11.5 Monitoring of IIH

- Whilst most patients follow a benign course, regular assessment of symptoms and visual function is necessary to identify those at risk of visual loss. No predictors of outcome have been identified, and the duration of IIH varies widely.
- Recurrence is not unusual.
  - Visual fields are the most sensitive test—arrange regular perimetry.
  - Regular measurement of CSF pressure is not useful, but a repeat LP may be indicated in cases of sudden deterioration, particularly when surgical intervention is being considered.
  - Advise patients to report worsening of their symptoms promptly and encourage persistence with attempts to lose weight.
- In most patients, recovery or remission will occur, but a small subgroup develop chronic symptoms, of which persistent headache is the most difficult to treat. 5% develop blindness in one or both eyes as optic atrophy develops.

Intracranial hypotension

Low pressure headache is brought on or aggravated by assuming the erect posture and relieved on assuming the horizontal posture. Because it may occur with apparently normal CSF pressures, loss of CSF volume may be responsible for the features.

Clinical features

There are two main types of low pressure headache:
- Post-lumbar puncture headache (dural puncture)
  - Occurs in about 1/3 of subjects undergoing diagnostic LP and about 1/5 undergoing obstetric procedures. About 90% of cases develop within 3 days of the procedure.
  - There tends to be one or more of neck stiffness, tinnitus, hyperacusis, photophobia or nausea. Most cases resolve spontaneously within 1 week, or within 48h of effective treatment, but 7% of subjects can be impaired for longer than this.
  - Earlier onset usually indicates a more severe and prolonged course.
- Spontaneous intracranial hypotension (SIH)
  - Incidence is 5 per 100 000 per year
  - The causes of spontaneous dural tears causing low pressure headache is not clear.
  - Meningeal diverticulae have been demonstrated intra-operatively in 40% of patients.
  - Connective tissue abnormalities have been suggested as possible underlying predisposing conditions following reports in patients with Marfan and Ehlers–Danlos syndromes.
  - Case reports have suggested that SIH may result from abnormalities of the cervical spine and chiropractic manoeuvres.
  - Has been reported after Valsalva manoeuvre, weight lifting and orgasm.
  - There is a high misdiagnosis rate of SIH of ~94%, and this results in diagnostic delays that could be as long as 13 years.
  - SIH can be complicated by venous sinus thrombosis resulting in loss of the postural pattern of the headache.
  - The onset of headache following SIH may be gradual or subacute. It has been known to present as a new daily headache.

Table 11.6 Risk factors for post-lumbar puncture headache

- More likely with larger, traumatic spinal needles but not with volume of CSF drained.
- More likely if the initial opening pressure is low.
- More common in young, thin females.
- Risk is less in the extremes of age and in subjects with dementia.
- Patients reporting headache before LP more likely to report post-LP headaches.

Table 11.7 Prevention of post-lumbar puncture headache

- Use of smaller gauge (22G) spinal needles
- Use of atraumatic spinal needles
- Directing the bevel of the needle horizontally
- Replacing the stylet and rotating the needle by 90° before withdrawal

The following have not been shown to be of benefit in prevention

- Imposed bed rest for up to 4h post-lumbar puncture
- Bed rest postures (supine, horizontal, prone, head-down tilt)
- Increased fluid intake
- Prophylactic paracetamol–caffeine combinations

Investigation of low pressure headache

Post-lumbar puncture headache usually does not need investigations because the clear temporal association with LP is sufficient to establish the diagnosis. The following investigations may be indicated in patients with SIH.

- Contrast MRI. This is usually the first investigation and shows several possible indices of low pressure:
  - Contrast enhancement of the meninges in >80%
  - Tonsillar descent in >40%
  - Subdural hygromas/haematomas in 17%
  - Dilated internal vertebral venous plexus in 85%
  - Spinal hygromas in 70%
  - Extrathecal CSF and haemosiderin as pointers of CSF leak

However, MRI can be normal
- Radioisotope cisternography
  - In more than half of cases, this shows the site of CSF leakage. Most of these are at the cervico-thoracic junction or thoracic spine.
  - Indirect markers of CSF leak are limited ascent of the tracer to the cerebral convexity, early appearance of radioisotope in the bladder and early soft tissue uptake of radioisotope.
  - The false-negative rate is 30%.
- CT myelography. This is the choice investigation to demonstrate the site of CSF leak.
  - Plain CT may show small ventricles and poorly visualized cerebral sulci.
  - In patients with complicated or multiple leaks, dynamic CT myelography may be more informative.
- Lumbar puncture
  - The opening pressure is typically low (0–5cm CSF) but is normal in up to 17% of cases.
  - LP can interfere with the interpretation of MRI findings and should be done only if other findings are equivocal.
  - High CSF protein and lymphocytic pleocytosis have been reported in a small number of cases.
- Colour Doppler flow imaging of the superior ophthalmic vein shows a larger vessel with a higher flow velocity which reverses with treatment.

Pathophysiology

- CSF leakage following a dural tear or puncture is the underlying mechanism of low pressure headache. The resultant loss of CSF volume causes traction on pain-sensitive structures that also support the brain—the meninges, the cerebral and cerebellar veins, the fifth, ninth and tenth cranial nerves, and the upper 3 cervical nerves.
- Compensatory cerebral vasodilatation occurs in an attempt to maintain CSF volume.
- These two mechanisms are thought to result in the headache. Assumption of the upright posture exacerbates these processes.

Table 11.8 Commonly associated clinical features in SIH

- Neck stiffness
- Tinnitus
- Hyperacusis
- Photophobia
- Nausea
- Interscapular pain
- Radicular upper limb pain
- Vertigo
- Visual field defects
- Cranial nerve palsies

Table 11.9 Rarely reported associated features in SIH

- Sudden deafness
- Orthostatic tinnitus
- Rapid onset encephalopathy and coma
- Parkinsonism
- Chorea
- Bipolar disorder
- Chronic behavioural features suggestive of frontotemporal dementia

Treatment of low pressure headache

In patients with severe symptoms, recurrent leaks occur in 28% of cases following treatment and almost always following surgical repair. Treatment of SIH may be complicated by development of intracranial hypertension.

- Conservative measures
  - Bed rest
  - Increased fluid intake
  - In a long-term follow-up of 13 patients with SIH treated conservatively, six still had mild to moderate headache 2 years afterwards, while recurrence occurred in one.
- Methylxanthines
  - IV caffeine, and to a much lesser extent theophylline, are used for non-response to conservative measures.
  - Thought to work by blocking adenosine receptors, causing vasoconstriction.
  - Caffeine is given at a dose of 500mg in 500ml saline over 2h.
  - There is a need to exclude arrhythmias.
- Autologous blood patch
  - Works via a tamponade effect.
  - Effective, and relief is typically immediate.
  - Effect spreads beyond the site of application up to about 4 intervertebral spaces. Because of this, blood patching does not have to be targeted to the site of the leak.
  - Consider early in high-risk subjects (age <50 years, post-partum, large-gauge needle puncture) and in severe cases.
- Surgery
  - This is usually resorted to if blood patch fails.
  - Consists of ligation of diverticulae or packing of epidural space with muscle or gel foam.
  - Post-surgery, complete relief is the rule, with no recurrence after 19-months follow-up.
  - It is not always possible to identify the site of leak intra-operatively even if myelography demonstrates one.
  - Surgery is not indicated for SDHs following SIH as they do not respond satisfactorily to drainage and resolve only with treatment of the leak.
- Other non-surgical therapies
  - Oral prednisolone, abdominal binders, epidural saline or dextran and fibrin sealant have been used successfully.

Headache associated with exertion, cough and sex

Introduction

Almost all headaches are worsened by exercise, or trigger a preference for rest or exertion (see Table 12.1).

Headaches may be triggered by cough, exertion and sex. The majority are primary where no underlying cause can be identified and where spontaneous remission is common. Studies report that 10–40% of cases are secondary where there is an identifiable pathology.

Mechanism of exertional headache

- Primary headache. Mechanisms are unknown but may include:
  - Recruitment of pain pathways
  - Disequilibration of intraspinal and intracerebral pressure at the foramen magnum.
  - Muscle damage resulting from straining
  - Venous distension
- Secondary exertional headache is caused by:
  - CSF obstruction due to cerebellar tonsillar ectopia (Chiari malformation) or, less commonly, a colloid cyst of the third ventricle
  - Tumour
  - SAH
  - Arterial dissection

(See Table 12.3.)

Cough headache

Primary cough headache is the exemplar of Valsalva-induced headache triggered by cough, sneeze, laughing, stooping or any other form of straining.
- Sudden onset lasting 1s to 30min
- Sharp or stabbing quality but dull pain may persist for hours
- Average age of onset 55 years
- Usually bilateral
- Treatment
  - Cough suppression
  - Indometacin 25–50 tds.
  - Some patients have prolonged relief following an LP
- Secondary cough headache is characterized by
  - Younger patient
  - Usually bilateral
  - Seconds to days duration
  - Can be precipitated by head or postural change

Table 12.1 The effect of exertion on other headaches

- Migraine is characteristically worsened by light exercise, with an almost universal preference for rest.
- In exercise-induced migraine there may be a delay of minutes or hours between exercise and migraine.
- Cluster headache usually makes the patient active, though activity does not normally improve the pain.
- Tension-type headache can be improved.

Table 12.2 Investigating exertional headache

- A primary headache can only be diagnosed in the absence of a secondary pathology. Neuroimaging is indicated for all first presentations.
- The first explosive headache occurring with any type should be investigated with CT and LP
- >2 episodes without disability, and attacks lasting >1h are unlikely to be SAH.

Physical exertion headache

- Primary headache
  - Most common
  - Brought on by physical exertion
  - Minutes to 48h
  - Pulsitile
  - Younger, 10–48 years
  - Usually bilateral
- Treatment:
  - Progressive exercise with warm up
  - Indometacin 25–50 tds
  - Propranolol 40mg 30min before exercise
  - Ergotamine 1–2mg or methylsergide 1–2mg orally 30min before exercise
- Secondary headache
  - Lasts longer—days to months
  - Can be explosive.

Headache associated with sexual activity

Classification is:
- Pre-orgasmic
  - Dull and bilateral
  - Increases with sexual excitement
- Orgasmic
  - Explosive headache
  - Occurs at orgasm
  - Studies report 4.5–12% caused by SAH
- Postural low CSF headache.
- Treatment of primary sex headache:
  - Sexual technique: relaxation, passive position, avoidance of multiple or serial orgasm. Contested treatment
  - Indometacin 25–75mg in anticipation of trigger
  - β-Blockers, taken either regularly or in single dose in anticipation of trigger—but may reduce libido!
  - Avoidance of drugs triggering headache: sildenafil and related drugs, recreational stimulants (cocaine, amphetamines, amyl nitrate)

Table 12.3 Structures implicated in exertional headache

Cerebellar tonsillar ectopia (Arnold–Chiari malformation)

- A structural abnormality in which the lower part of the cerebellum, the tonsils, protrude through the foramen magnum into the spinal subarachnoid space.
- Minor degrees of this are not uncommon
- The greater the cerebellar descent, and the more crowded the structures at the foramen magnum, the greater the chance of the lesion being significant and in need of surgical treatment—foramen magnum decompression.
- This lesion is sometimes complicated by syringomyelia, often though not inevitably causing paraparesis and sensory change including arm pain. The presence of a syrinx provides strong if not compelling indication for surgery.
- Other clinical features of cerebellar tonsillar ectopia may include downbeating nystagmus and a C2/3 pinprick level

Colloid cyst of the third ventricle

- Relatively uncommon.
- Can present with acute hydrocephalus causing attacks of unconsciousness and sudden death.
- Occasional incidental finding on brain imaging, sometimes seen better on CT than on MRI, where it can be overlooked.
- The optimal management without hydrocephalus is uncertain and challenging.

Intracerebral mass lesions

- Rarely present with exertional headache.
- Mechanisms include hydrocephalus, downward displacement of hindbrain structures causing cerebellar tonsillar ectopia, midline shift and non-specific pressure effects.
- There are usually features other than headache including seizures, papilloedema, impaired consciousness or cognition, and upper motor neuron signs in the limbs.

Other secondary headaches

Headaches attributed to vascular disorders

Headaches due to stroke

Transient ischaemic attack

- Headaches are reported in 16–36% of patients with TIAs.
- The cause of headaches in TIA is uncertain, but they usually occur on the same side as that of the TIA and are more common with a carotid territory event.
- Migraine with aura is the main differential diagnosis in patients with headache associated with TIA. The speed of onset and resolution of the neurological deficit, previous history of similar attacks, family history and negative diagnostic work up point to the diagnosis.
- Antiphospholipid antibody syndrome, cerebral AVM, neoplasm and expanding vascular aneurysm may also present with headache and focal neurological deficits.

Ischaemic stroke

- The cause of headaches in ischaemic stroke is unknown.
- It is less common then haemorrhagic stroke.
- May be under-reported due to concurrent severe neurological deficits and presence of speech impairment and altered mentation.
- More pronounced with a posterior circulation event.
- Headache does not correlate with location or size of the infarct though more pronounced with large artery strokes.
- Headache may have abrupt or gradual onset, usually unilateral, mild to moderate in intensity and non-specific in character, with nausea. Vomiting and photophobia are uncommon.

Haemorrhagic stroke

- Between 33 and 65% of patients report headaches.
- More common in women, those with cerebellar bleed, tentorial herniation, mass effect and signs of meningeal herniation.
- The majority of patients have unilateral focal headache depending upon location of the haematoma. Intraventricular haemorrhage causes a diffuse headache. The character is non-specific, with vomiting in around half of the patients.
- Putamenial bleed is associated with ipsilateral frontal headache, while occipital headaches indicate cerebellar or occipital bleed.

Table 13.1 HS-coded headaches attributed to cranial or cervical vascular disorders

- Headache attributed to ischaemic stroke or TIA
  - Ischaemic stroke
  - TIA
- Headache attributed to non-traumatic intracranial haemorrhage
  - Intracerebral haemorrhage
  - SAH
- Headache attributed to unruptured vascular malformation
  - Saccular aneurysm
  - AVM
  - Arteriovenous fistula
  - Cavernous angioma
- Headache attributed to arteritis
  - Giant cell arteritis
  - Central nervous system angiitis
- Carotid or vertebral artery pain
- Headache attributed to cerebral venous thrombosis
- Headache attributed to other intracranial vascular disorder
  - Cerebral autosomal dominant arteriopathy with subcortical infarcts and leukoencephalopathy
  - Mitochondrial encephalopathy, lactic acidosis and stroke-like symptoms
  - Benign angiopathy of the CNS
  - Pituitary apoplexy

Headaches related to unruptured vascular malformations

- Prevalence of incidental and asymptomatic aneurysm 3–6%.
- Multiple aneurysms (usually 2–3) occur in ~20% of patients. This strongly correlates with hypertension.
- Vast majority of these never rupture or cause any symptoms.
- Rarely unruptured aneurysms may produce warning symptoms including headaches because of either impending rupture or progressive enlargement leading to compression of neighbouring structures.
- The annual incidence of rupture of incidental aneurysms <7mm is 0.1%, and 1.5% in those between 7 and 12mm.
- Unruptured AVMs may produce headaches mimicking migraine. If they bleed, they usually present as seizures or intraparenchymal haemorrhage.

Headaches associated with carotid or vertebral dissection

- Dissection and/or occlusion of the internal carotid artery causes unilateral headache.
- May be associated with ipsilateral Horner's syndrome with contralateral neurological signs or symptoms.
- The pain can involve head, neck or face. Vertebral artery dissection causes pain in the upper neck and occiput, and may be associated with lateral medullary syndrome or cerebellar infarction.

Headaches due to arteritis

- Giant cell arteritis (temporal arteritis) is the most commonest cause of arteritis. Recent onset of new headaches in patients above the age of 50 should alert the physician (see Table 13.2).
- Systemic disease, e.g. SLE.
- CNS angiitis
  - Primary or secondary
  - Encephalic signs, e.g. stroke, fit, disorders of cognition or consciousness
  - Can be angiographic signs,

Table 13.2 Clinical features of giant cell arteritis

Epidemiology

- Rarely reported in patients younger then 50 years beyond which the incidence rises dramatically with age.
- Rare in Asians and Afro-Americans and is specially common in persons of British and Scandinavian origin.
- Twice as common in women.

Symptoms

- Headaches; uni- or bitemporal, often throbbing or burning with head soreness or cutaneous allodynia (sensitivity to touch, brushing, combing, etc.).
- Jaw claudication—an aching in the jaw or temporalis muscle on chewing
- Constitutional symptoms. Anorexia, recent weight loss, insomnia, fever, night sweats and malaise
- Pain and aching in shoulder and less often pelvic girdle muscles indicate accompanying polymyalgia rheumatica.

Signs

- Tender, non-pulsatile or beaded temporal artery
- Pallor of optic disc with associated ischaemic optic neuropathy
- Often signs are absent

Diagnosis

- Clinical suspicion
- ESR/PV is raised in the majority of patients (1–2% may be normal)
- CRP is raised. This is equally sensitive but more specific than ESR and is more useful parameter for diagnosing and monitoring disease activity.
- Temporal artery biopsy is helpful if conducted before or within 48h of commencing steroid treatment. It may be normal because of skip areas of vascular pathology or because giant cell arteritis may affect other cranial vessels without involving temporal arteries.

Treatment

- Responds dramatically and rapidly with high dose steroid therapy (prednisolone 60–80mg/day).
- The dose is tapered slowly over 6–12 months, although many patients require a low dose steroid for many years.
- Immunosuppression has little role as a steroid-sparing stategy
- Monitoring is done with regular measurement of ESR and CRP, and recurrence of symptoms when the dose of steroid is decreased

Complications

- If untreated may result in visual loss
- The time between first symptom and visual loss varies from a few weeks to a few months.

Headache due to cerebral venous thrombosis
Epidemiology
- The exact incidence is unknown owing to its varied presentation.
- Affects all age groups although common in the 3rd and 4th decade with a male:female ratio of 1:3. Predisposing conditions are shown in Table 13.5.
- Women of childbearing age and those on oral contraceptive pill or smokers are at a high risk.

Diagnosis
- Maintain a high index of suspicion especially in cases with high risk of venous thrombosis.
- Gradual onset of diffuse, continuous and progressive headache.
- Retro-orbital pain in cases of cavernous sinus or lateral sinus thrombosis.
- Focal symptoms, e.g. facial numbness, focal seizures, double vision, indicate cortical vein thrombosis.
- Features of raised intracranial pressure with drowsiness, visual blurring and postural headache may develop with time.
- Signs of raised intracranial pressure: papilloedema, 6th nerve palsy, clouding of consciousness
- Focal neurological signs indicating cortical thrombosis
- Proptosis and ophthalmoparesis in cavernous sinus thrombosis.

Investigation
- MRI and MRV are the best imaging for diagnosis, although CT scan may show the empty triangle sign.
- CSF examination may help in excluding meningitis and encephalitis, and may be therapeutic in relieving headache due to raised intracranial pressure.
- Routine blood tests including autoimmune profile, thrombophilia screen, antiphospholipid antibody, serum electrophoresis may reveal an underlying cause.

Rare but important vascular headaches (see Chapter 4)
CADISIL
- Migraine with or without aura without other neurological signs.
- Typical white matter changes on MRI.
- Diagnostic confirmation from skin biopsy or genetic testing.
- Recurrent small deep infarcts, subcortical dementia and mood disturbances.

MELAS
- Attacks of migraine with or without aura.
- Stroke-like episodes and seizures.
- Genetic abnormality.

Headache attributed to pituitary apoplexy
- Severe headache with clinical and neuroimaging evidence of acute haemorrhagic pituitary infarction.
- Acute and life threatening.
- Can present as thunderclap headache.

Table 13.3 Treatment of headache due to cerebral venous thrombosis

- Anticoagulation is the standard accepted therapy
- IV heparin should be commenced immediately and continued until the APTT is twice the pre-treatment level or until resolution of acute symptoms, e.g. headache, seizures, drowsiness
- Warfarin should be commenced and be continued for 6 months or indefinitely in those with underlying coagulopathy
- Role of thrombolysis is unclear due to lack of randomized trials, and its routine use is not recommended
- Anticonvulsants if seizures occur
- Diuretics for raised intracranial pressure, e.g. acetazolamide
- Steroids and immunosuppressants in those with autoimmune conditions

Table 13.4 Prognosis of headache due to cerebral venous thrombosis

- Prognosis is usually favourable
- Mortality rate <20% and often as low as 4%
- Main causes of death are massive stroke, seizures, sepsis, pulmonary embolism or underlying malignancy
- Poor prognosis is seen in those with focal neurological signs including seizures, rapid onset of coma and extremes of age
- The most common residual symptom is seizure and headache, occurring in 10% cases

Table 13.5 Predisposing conditions for cerebral venous thrombosis

Genetic conditions
- Protein S, protein C deficiency
- Antithrombin 3 deficiency
- Homocystinuria

Acquired conditions
- Pregnancy, puperium, oral contraceptive pills, rarely HRT
- Antiphospholipid antibody syndrome
- Thrombocytosis
- Polycythaemia
- Previous deep venous thrombosis,
- Pulmonary embolism or cerebral venous thrombosis
- Neoplastic conditions, e.g. leukaemia, lymphoma
- Infective conditions, e.g. otitis media, mastoiditis
- Injury to dural sinus; surgery trauma
- Inflammatory conditions, e.g. Behcet's disease, ulcerative colitis

Headaches due to systemic or metabolic diseases (disorders of homeostasis)

Headaches at high altitude

- A rapid ascent to high altitude can produce acute mountain sickness.
- Moderate to severe diffuse headaches with nausea, fatigue, dizziness and sleep disturbance.
- Attributed to hypoxia, but changes in fluid and electrolytes may play a part.
- Is more common in people with primary headache disorders.
- Diuretics such as spironolactone and acetazolamide may be used as preventative treatment.

Headaches associated with diving

- May be a component of decompression sickness, arterial gas embolism, otic barotraumas or related to hypercapnia and/or carbon monoxide toxicity.
- Headaches are diffuse and associated with other features of hypercapnia including confusion, dyspnoea, flushed face, flapping tremor followed by cardiorespiratory depression, convulsion and loss of consciousness.

Headaches associated with carbon monoxide poisoning

- Headache is an early symptom of carbon monoxide poisoning.
- Associated with dizziness, dyspnoea and nausea.
- Due to hypoxia once carboxyhaemoglobin level exceeds 15%.
- Treatment of carbon monoxide poisoning is inhalation of 100% oxygen or hyperbaric oxygen to speed carboxyhaemoglobin dissociation.

Headaches due to obstructive sleep apnoea

- Commonly affects overweight men.
- Characterized by loud snoring and apnoeac spells that produce restless sleep during the night followed by early morning headache and day time sleepiness and tiredness.
- Confirmed with overnight sleep oximetry.
- Patients should be encouraged to lose weight, stop smoking, and avoid sedative or excessive alcohol and sleep deprivation.
- Treatment with the use of intranasal continuous positive air pressure (CPAP) improves symptoms.

Dialysis headaches

- 70% of patients receiving haemodialysis complain of frontal headaches either of tension type or throbbing with nausea and vomiting.
- Starts within a few hours of the procedure and is proportional to time spent on dialysis.
- Hypertension, hypotension during procedure, hypoxaemia, hyponatraemia, reduced serum osmolality, changes in urea and aldosterone and release of vasoactive peptide are thought to be the precipitating cause.

Hypoglycaemia and fasting headaches

- Can produce headaches similar to migraines or typically produces migraine in susceptible individuals.
- Can occur if meals are missed. Fasting is associated with non-pulsating continuous bilateral diffuse or frontal headache which is directly proportional to the duration of fast, usually occurring after 16h.
- More common in patients with primary headache disorder and may not be related to hypoglycaemia. Dehydration may also play a part.
- Headache can occur with glucose intolerance ~2h after the meal.

Headaches in phaeochromocytoma

- Catecholamine-producing tumours that arise from chromaffin cells. Usually in the adrenal medulla but can occur in extra-adrenal tissues.
- Headaches are often frontal or occipital, pulsating but usually last <1h.
- Associated with sweating, anxiety, nausea, tremor, pallor and palpitation. Majority of patients have hypertension.
- Diagnosis is increased excretion of metanephrine, normetanephrine, vinylmandelic acid and total catecholamine in 24h urine sample.
- Drug treatment is usually with an α-1 adrenergic blocker.

Headaches and hypertension

- The subject is contested. Mild hypertension does not cause headache and there is little evidence for moderate hypertension.
- Abrupt and severe rise in blood pressure may be associated with headaches.
- Hypertensive encephalopathy is caused by sudden, severe hypertension
  - Is characterzed by headaches, nausea, vomiting, visual disturbance, altered mental status, seizures and focal neurological deficits.
  - MRI abnormalities of posterior white matter oedema in parietal and occipital lobes and brainstem.
  - Complete recovery occurs with prompt treatment.

Hyperthyroidism and headaches

- Headache is mild, bilateral, continuous non-pulsating, with nausea, vomiting and sensitivity to light and sound.
- Responds within 2 weeks of hormone therapy.
- More common in patients with primary headache disorders.

Headaches with pre-eclampsia and eclampsia

- Characterized by a triad of hypertension, oedema and protienuria occurring beyond 20 weeks of gestation. Eclampsia is the occurrence of seizure with or without pre-eclampsia.
- Headaches occurring in both conditions are bilateral pulsating and exacerbated with physical activity. Sudden headaches have also been described.

Cardiac cephalalgia
- Headaches occurring at the same time as cardiac ischaemia. Important to distinguish from migraine without aura as triptans are contraindicated in ischaemic heart disease.
- Glyceryl trinitrate spray given for treatment of angina also produces vascular headaches.

Hot dog headaches
- Due to nitrites added to salt to give uniform red appearance to cured meat.

Chinese restaurant syndrome
- Monosodium glutamate used in Chinese recipes can cause tension-type or migraine-like headaches.
- 15–20min after eating a Chinese meal.

Headache associated with psychiatric disorders
- Can be due to the psychiatric disorder, associated stress or medication taken for treatment.
- Headache attributed to a psychiatric disorder is only definitive if it remits following successful treatment of the disorder.
- Unipolar depression.
  - Migraine is three times more common in patients with depression, and depression is five times more prevalent with migraine. SSRIs may cause headaches.
  - The headache in unipolar depression is more frequently right sided.
- Bipolar disorders
  - These are often left sided.
  - Migraine is more common in patients with bipolar disorders.
  - Patients are often younger and more educated and have few psychiatric hospitalizations.
  - Sodium valproate is the treatment of choice for when migraine is co-morbid.
- Anxiety disorders. Headaches are more common in panic disorders, generalized anxiety, phobias and post-traumatic stress disorder, although the link between these disorders and headaches is not strong.
- Psychotic disorders. Headache in schizophrenia is similar to that of the general population.

Headaches associated with CNS infection

Meningitis

Meningitis implies serious infection of the meninges. This is a medical emergency and requires immediate referral to specialist care. Acute bacterial meningitis has 15% mortality even with optimal care.

Causes

These may be infective, infiltrative, reaction to blood in ventricles and subarachnoid space, and drugs. Common infective causes are given in Table 13.6.

Symptoms

These are less pronounced in viral meningitis.

- Recent onset of diffuse, progressive and often pulsating headaches
- Nausea, vomiting
- Intense photo- and phonophobia
- Fever with rigors and malaise
- Neck pain and stiffness
- Altered level of consciousness, confusion

Signs

- Patient is irritable and prefers to lie still
- Fever
- Delirium and drowsiness which is progressive
- Neck rigidity
- Kernig's sign
- Lateralizing signs
- In meningococcal infection, petechial rash

Diagnosis

- Recognize and treat early.
- CT scan should be done before lumbar puncture in cases with symptoms or signs of raised intracranial pressure.
- CSF examination provides essential information to the underlying cause. See Table 13.7.
- CSF must be sent for microbial identification.

Treatment

- Start immediately with benzylpenicillin 1200mg slow IV or IM prior to LP results.
- Cefotaxime 1g IV is an alternative in those with penicillin allergy.

Chronic meningitis

- Typically TB or fungal.
- Patient is unwell for some weeks if not months.
- Vague headaches, fever often low grade, anorexia, malaise.
- Focal neurological signs such as papilloedema and seizure may develop.

Table 13.6 Infective causes of meningitis

- Bacterial
  - *Neisseria meningitidis*
  - *Streptococcus pneumoniae*
  - *Staphylococcus aureus*
  - Group B *Streptococcus*
  - *Listeria monocytogenes*
  - *Escherichia coli*
  - *Haemophilus influenzae*
  - *Borrelia burgdorferi*
  - *Mycobacterium tuberculosis*
- Viral
  - Herpes simplex
  - Mumps
  - Enteroviruses, e.g. Coxsackie, ECHO
  - Epstein–Barr virus
  - JC virus
  - HIV
- Fungal
  - *Cryptococcus neformans*
  - *Candida*

Table 13.7 CSF changes in meningitis

	Viral	Pyogenic	Tuberculosis
Appearance	Clear/turbid	Turbid/purulent	Turbid/viscous
Protein	<1g/l	1–2g/l	1–3g/l
Glucose	<1/2 blood glucose	>1/2blood glucose	>1/2 blood glucose
Mononuclears	10–100/mm^3	<50/mm^3	100–300/mm^3
Polymorphs	Few seen early	200–300/mm^3	0–200/mm^3

Encephalitis

Encephalitis is inflammation of brain parenchyma and is usually viral, although bacterial and fungal infection may be implicated. Many infections are mild and full recovery occurs.

Symptoms
- Fever
- Headaches
- Mood changes
- Confusion
- Seizures

Signs
- Fever
- Drowsiness
- Focal signs

Investigations
- CT and MRI often shows diffuse oedema in the temporal lobes.
- EEG often shows slow waves over the affected areas.
- CSF picture is similar to viral meningitis. PCR is mostly positive in HSV-1 infection.
- Viral serology is also helpful.

Treatment
- HSV infection is treatable and hence in suspected cases IV aciclovir should be commenced immediately.
- Poor outlook in patients presenting with coma.
- Anticonvulsants should be given in those with seizures.

Brain abscess/subdural empyema

- May occur secondary to skull fracture, paranasal, teeth or middle ear infection.
- Symptoms are more gradual in onset with focal neurological signs.
- Fever, leukocytosis and raised ESR is usual.
- Urgent imaging is required. LP is dangerous and unhelpful.
- Treatment is infection specific, and neurosurgical intervention may be required.

Headaches attributed to systemic infection

- Headache is a non-specific symptom and is usually diffuse, moderate to severe and associated with fever, malaise and laboratory evidence of infection.
- Migraine and TTHs can be precipitated or worsened with systemic infections.

It is often difficult to differentiate between headache in response to systemic infection or a result of a CNS infection. CSF examination is often required, especially in the presence of other neurological sign and symptoms.

Chapter 14

Medication overuse headache

Introduction

Medication overuse headache is headache that occurs on ≥15 days a month associated with frequent use of acute relief medication in susceptible patients. Patients with a migrainous predisposition seem prone to medication overuse headache. Acute relief medication alone does not cause headache in patients who do not have this susceptibility.

Epidemiology

The population prevalence is 1–2% and all age groups are affected.

Clinical features

- The headache should resolve or return to its previous pattern within ~2 months after discontinuation of the overused medication.
  - Patients with TTH as their primary headache develop chronic daily headache with the clinical syndrome of chronic TTH.
  - Patients with migraine headache as their primary headache develop either chronic TTH, daily migraine headache or an increased frequency of migraine attacks.
  - Patients with CH do not seem prone to the development of increased frequency of cluster attacks with frequent acute-relief medication use. However, there is a subgroup of patient who do develop medication overuse headache. These patients have either a past or a family history of migraine. The clinical picture of the medication overuse headache is either a daily TTH or migraine.
- HC patients can also develop medication overuse headache.
- All acute-relief medications have been implicated in medication overuse headache (Table 14.1).
- The delay between frequent medication intake and the development of medication overuse headache is shortest with the triptans (1.7 years), longer for ergots (2.7 years) and longest for analgesics (4.8 years).
- The frequency of days that acute-relief medication is taken is more important than the total dose consumption.
- The acute withdrawal period, during which patients can experience rebound headache, lasts ~10 days. Improvement thereafter can take 6–12 weeks and occurs gradually.
- Preventative medication is not adequately efficacious in the presence of medication overuse

Pathology

The mechanism of development of medication overuse headache is not known.

Table 14.1 Acute-relief medications reported in association with medication overuse headache

- NSAIDs
- Paracetamol
- Caffeine
- Ergotamine derivatives
- Opioid analgesics
- Triptans

Table 14.2 IHS classification criteria of critical frequencies of acute-relief medication use in medication overuse headache

- Ergotamine on ≥10 days of the month for at least 3 months.
- Triptan intake ≥10 days of the month for at least 3 months.
- Simple analgesics on ≥5 days of the month for at least 3 months.

Treatment

- Treatment recommendations for drug withdrawal vary and are based mainly on open label studies.
- Community or outpatient withdrawal is recommended for highly motivated patients who are adequately supported. The patient should be ready to change and may require support for sick leave. They should also be warned of potential withdrawal effects apart from worsening of headache (Table 14.3).
- There is a higher risk of psychiatric disorders in patients with chronic headache, particularly chronic migraine associated with substance overuse. Patients with medication overuse headache and psychiatric co-morbidity do less well.
- Anxiety and depression should be managed prior to withdrawal.

Community withdrawal

- Reported beneficial withdrawal regimens for primary/intermediate care are shown in Table 14.4.

Inpatient withdrawal

- Inpatient approaches include the use of IV dihydroergotamine, IV aspirin, IM chlorpromazine and IV lidocaine.
- The original IV dihydroergotamine protocol runs over 3½ days and requires inpatient monitoring over this time. The most common side effect is nausea in about 1/3 patients. An 8hrly 1mg protocol, up to 10mg total dose, with antiemetic pre-emptively can be used. Options for the latter include domperidone, metoclopramide or granisetron. Other common adverse effects include tightness and burning, leg cramps, vomiting and increased blood pressure.
- IV aspirin 1000mg can be given 8–12hrly.
- Parenteral chlorpromazine 12.5–25mg 3–4 times daily during withdrawal can provide pain relief, sedation and antiemetic effects. The maximum 24h recommended dose is 150mg. The main adverse effects include drowsiness and postural hypotension.
- The use of clonidine can be indicated for patients who develop opioid withdrawal (sweating, diarrhoea, pupillary dilation).

Table 14.3 Common effects following drug withdrawal of acute-relief medication (from the pre-triptan era)

- Vomiting 68%
- Nausea 39%
- Insomnia 36%
- Sweating 35%
- Anxiety and unsteadiness 30%
- Tachycardia 19%
- Tremor 13%
- Vertigo 12%
- Hallucinations 7%
- Nightmares 4%

Table 14.4 Community drug withdrawal

- Choose a suitable time for withdrawal and ensure patient is adequately supported .
- The acute withdrawal period can be covered with prednisolone 1mg/kg over 1 week tapered thereafter over 2 weeks, or naproxen 500mg bd during the first 2 weeks. The use of the latter has been based on lack of associated data with medication overuse headache, but this may reflect infrequent use of this drug. Use of alternative NSAIDs has been associated with headache recurrence within 6–8.
- Introduce preventative treatment following withdrawal if the patient is still experiencing >4-5 headache days/month.

Prognosis of treated medication overuse headache

- A successful response (>50% reduction in headache) is obtained in 60–80% of individuals.
- This rate plateaus by 12–24 months after withdrawal.
- Over time the relapse rate is 40%.
- Patients with migraine do better than those with TTH or a combination of disorders
- Triptan overusers do better than analgesic overusers.

Headache in children

Introduction

Headache is one of the most common complaints in children. Around 3 in 4 schoolchildren complain of headache at least once a year. 1 in 4 complains of at least 3 attacks of headache that are severe enough to interfere with normal activity.

Secondary headache

- Acute-onset secondary headache.
  - A common feature of many systemic illnesses including upper respiratory tract infection, otitis media, gastroenteritis and non-specific viral illnesses.
  - A consistent symptom in children with meningitis, but the clinical picture is dominated with other more serious symptoms pointing to the diagnosis.
  - Can be associated with recurrent illness e.g. to children with asthma.
- Chronic secondary headache
  - Benign underlying conditions such as constipation
  - Serious neurological disorder such as a brain tumour or raised intracranial pressure. Other symptoms and signs are almost always present to aid in the diagnosis.

Primary headache

Migraine

Epidemiology

- Migraine is the most common cause of severe recurrent headache.
- Prevalence rate of 10.6% in schoolchildren between 5 and 15 years of age.
- Increasing from 3.4% at age 5 to a peak of 19.1% at age 12 years (Fig. 15.1).
- During early childhood, girls and boys are equally affected, but after the age of 12 years, migraine is more common in girls than in boys (Fig. 15.2).
- Onset at any age from early infancy with two distinct peaks observed at age 5 and 12 years (Fig. 15.3).
- Migraine affects children from all social, economic and racial backgrounds and is a global problem.

Clinical features

- The main differences between childhood migraine and migraine in adults is summarized in Table 15.1. Childhood disorders related to migraine are shown in Table 15.2. Some specific characteristics are:
- Trigger factors can be subtle and children have a low threshold to stress, missing meals, missing sleep and variation in climate and weather.

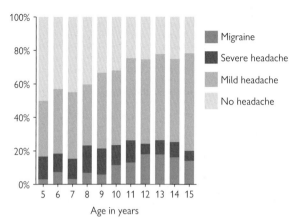

Fig. 15.1 Annual prevalence of headache and migraine in Aberdeen schoolchildren.

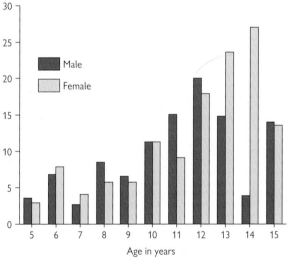

Fig. 15.2 Annual prevalence (%) of migraine among boys and girls 5–15 years.

- Short attacks of <2h are not uncommon. This phenomenon may exaggerate the placebo response to acute rescue treatment and increases the difficulties in interpreting RCTs of new and old therapies.
- It is difficult for children, especially those under the age of 8 years, to describe the quality of pain. Pain is often referred to as 'just sore' or 'can't describe.' Only a minority of children can describe the throbbing nature of headache.
- The location of maximum pain is often described as frontal, especially in young children.
- Unilateral headache becomes more prominent in adolescents and young adults.
- Severity of headache is best assessed by observing the behaviour of the younger child during attacks.
  - The child prefers to be left alone and to lie down or sleep in a darkened room.
  - Stops normal activities such as watching television, playing with toys and other children. Walking worsens symptoms.
  - Headache can be described as severe if the child stops all activities, moderate if they stop some but not all activities and mild if the child continues with normal daily activities despite the headache.
  - Child looks pale, unwell and most parents say that they can tell child is having a headache without the child telling them.
  - The child is reluctant to take normal meals, feels nauseated and may vomit.
  - Children gain comfort from rest, sleep and taking simple analgesics.
  - Between attacks the child is well and free of symptoms.

Management of headache. General principles

- Accurate diagnosis gives the family and the child confidence in treatment and removes doubts or anxiety about other sinister causes such as a brain tumour.
- If neuroimaging is indicated it should be done at early stages. Indications for neuroimaging in children with chronic headache are presented in Table 15.3.
- Non-pharmacological management of idiopathic headache is effective both in prevention and in treatment of headache attacks.
  - The child is encouraged to identify and avoid any possible trigger factors such as certain types of food, stress or anxiety.
  - Sedentary lifestyle, poor sleep routine, missing meal times, poor diet, anxiety and stressful life events increase the risk of headache.
  - Encourage an active healthy life style with good balance of regular exercise and rest.
  - Advise regular meals, healthy eating habits with a variety of food, drinking the appropriate amount of water and avoiding prolonged fasting or skipping meals, particularly breakfast.
  - Reduce the intake of caffeine-containing drinks.
  - A regular sleeping pattern and a predictable time for going to bed and for wakening up in the morning help in reducing headache frequency and severity.

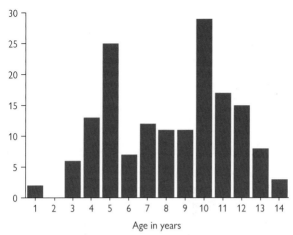

Fig. 15.3 Age of onset of migraine in 159 schoolchildren.

Table 15.1 Distinguishing features of childhood migraine compared with migraine in adult patients

	Childhood migraine	Migraine in adults
Duration of attacks	1–72h	4–72h
Description of headache	Often vague and not possible	Throbbing is common
Site of maximum pain	Frontal in at least 50%	Unilateral in the majority
Severity of pain	Manifested by change in behaviour	Well described
Measurement of image	School absenteeism	Time off work
Associated abdominal pain	Common	Rare

• Professional help from a clinical psychologist may improve the child's responses to pain, anxiety and stressful circumstances.
• Relaxation, biofeedback, CBT and other techniques can be helpful.

Migraine acute treatment (see Table 15.4)

● Only a small proportion of children seek medical advice. The majority are managed by their parents who may suffer from migraine and either are confident in the interpretation of symptoms and treatment or resigned to the misconception that there is no effective treatment.
● Successful treatment of migraine attacks depends on the recognition of early symptoms and the administration of the most appropriate painkiller in an appropriate dose and via the most appropriate route of administation.
● There is a tendency for parents and practitioners to administer small doses of analgesia and also to delay administration of treatment until headache is established and severe enough to warrant treatment.
● For effective pain relief, analgesics should be given in their optimum doses, 10–20mg/kg every 6–8h (maximum 60mg/kg/day) for paracetamol and 10–15mg/kg every 6–8h for Ibuprofen.
● In some children, nausea and vomiting are relatively early symptoms. Early treatment with antiemetic drugs such as cyclizine or metoclopramide may help and improve the response to pain killers.
● Sumatriptan or zolmitriptan is effective and can be indicated for children over the age of 12 years. Nasal sumatriptan in a dose of 10mg is shown to be effective and safe in adolescents.

Migraine preventative treatment (see Table 15.5)

● Prevention is indicated with frequent episodes of headache (at least 4 attacks per month), long attacks and when severe enough to interfere with the quality of life and education.
● Due to the natural course of migraine in children characterized by alternating spells of remissions and relapses, the placebo effect is often exaggerated, making the assessment of drug efficiency difficult to interpret.
● There is no ideal medicine that offers consistent results with minimal or no side effects.
● Pizotifen is commonly used for its safety, but the response rate is unpredictable.
● Propranolol can be useful in a dose of 2–3mg/kg/day.
● Other drugs include amitriptyline, topiramate and valproate are possible prophylactic agents.
● Preventative treatment should be used for at least 3 months in optimum dose before it can be judged as effective or unhelpful.

Tension type headache

Epidemiology

● Prevalence as defined by IHS criteria is 9.8% in 7- to 15-year-old schoolchildren, but rises to 23% on using unrestricted criteria.
● Male and females are equally affected and it is more common in older children.

Table 15.2 Childhood periodic syndromes (see Chapter 4)

Three childhood periodic syndromes are commonly precursors of migraine.
Their exact relationship to migraine remains contested.

- Cyclical vomiting
  - Recurrent episodic attacks of vomiting and intense nausea
  - Associated with power and lethargy
  - Lasts between 1h and 5 days
  - Are individually stereotypical
- Abdominal migraine
  - Episodic mid-line abdominal pain
  - Lasting 1–72h
  - Moderate to severe intensity
  - Can be associated with vasomotor symptoms, nausea and vomiting
  - Invariably interferes with normal daily activities
  - Most children will develop migraine later in life.
- Benign paroxysmal vertigo of childhood
  - Recurrent brief attacks of vertigo
  - Occurs without warning
  - Resolves spontaneously
  - Can last minutes to hours
  - Neurological examination and investigation is normal
  - Can be associated with nystagmus or vomiting
  - Unilateral headache may occur in association.

Table 15.3 Indications for neuroimaging in children with chronic headache

- Features of cerebellar dysfunction
  - Ataxia
  - Nystagmus
  - Intention tremor
- Features of increased intracranial pressure
  - Papilloedema
  - Night time or early morning headache and vomiting
  - Large head
- New focal neurological deficits including recent squint
- Seizures, especially focal
- Personality change
- Unexplained deterioration of school work

- TTH is rare in children under the age of 6 years.
- Chronic daily headache is relatively uncommon. Chronic TTH is the most common cause reported in 0.9% of schoolchildren.

Clinical features
- TTH is defined as frequent, infrequent or chronic in nature.
- Duration is usually short, but may be continuous in chronic TTH.
- Described as pressure or tightening and mild to moderate in severity.
- Bilateral in location and does not worsen with routine activities.
- May be associated with photophobia or phonophobia, but not nausea or vomiting.
- Diagnosis is made on the basis of the typical clinical history and normal neurological examination. Investigations are not needed in the majority of patients.
- Clinical features of TTH can sometimes be indistinguishable from those of migraine without aura, and the correct diagnosis is best made by the use of prospective headache diaries.
- In some patients, both migraine without aura and TTH co-exist. The distinction between the two conditions is important in order to plan treatment and predict outcome.

Management of TTH
- Can be complex and multidisciplinary.
- Should aim at reassuring the child and the parents of the absence of any sinister cause.
- Offer general advice on healthy lifestyle as above.
- Successful management will need the full involvement of the child, their parents, schoolteachers or nurses, and occasionally clinical psychologists.
- Attention should be paid to possible underlying chronic physical, psychological or emotional problems.
- Pharmacological treatment of acute attacks with simple analgesics is often effective and sufficient in infrequent TTH.
- Pharmacological treatment is largely unsuccessful, and analgesics should be discouraged in chronic TTH, as some may develop analgesia overuse headache on long-term use.
- Preventative treatment is occasionally needed to reduce distress caused by daily or almost daily attacks. Amitriptyline in dosages between 10 and 50mg/day (up to 1mg/kg/day) can be used.
- The prognosis of TTH is variable and patients may run a course of remissions and relapses.

Table 15.4 Medication used in acute treatment of migraine

Drug	Dose	
	Under 12 years	**12–18 years**
Paracetamol	10–20mg/kg Max 4 times/day	500–1000mg Max 4 times/day
Ibuprofen	10–15mg/kg Max 4 times/day	400mg Max 4 times/day
Diclofenac	3–5mg/kg/day Max 4 times/day	3–5mg/kg/day Max 4 times/day
Codeine	0.5–1.0mg/kg Max 4 times/day	30–60mg Max 4 times/day
Metoclopramide	100mcg/kg Max 3 times/day	2.5–10mg Max 4 times/day
Sumatriptan nasal spray		10mg Max twice/day

Table 15.5 Medication used in preventative treatment of migraine

Drug	Dose	
	Under 12 years	**12–18 years**
Pizotifen	0.5–1.0mg/day Single dose at night	1.5–3.0mg/day Single dose at night
Propranolol	0.2–0.5mg/kg Max 4.0mg/kg/day	2–3mg/kg/day Max 160mg/day
Amitriptyline		Up to 50mg/night
Topiramate		2–3mg/kg/day Gradual increase to target dose

Chapter 16

Headache in the elderly

Introduction

Although the prevalence of headache reduces with age, it remains a common problem (Table 16.1). More than 5% of the population over the age of 80 years have frequent headache.

Specific problems in the elderly

- Increase in co-morbidity and disease susceptibility. This has implications for treatment options.
- Polypharmacy. Often drugs can cause headache.
- Reduced renal and liver function leading to altered pharmokinetics. Increased vigilance is required when prescribing for headache.
- Increased risk of adverse drug reactions.
- Limited evidence base. Few studies have been undertaken in this age group.

Primary headache in the elderly

Cluster headache
- Less common but often remains undiagnosed.

Tension-type headache
- Although 10% of patients with TTH develop it after the age of 50, it becomes less prevalent. An association with medication overuse headache can make diagnosis problematic.

Migraine
In general, migraine has a favourable prognosis, with a decrease in prevalence from the age of 50 onwards in both sexes (see Fig 4.1).
- Prevalence rates remain at between 3 and 5% even over the age of 70.
- Migraine can develop after the age of 50, but onset is rare after the age of 60.
- Over the age of 50, 10% will have an abnormality on imaging, and investigations should be undertaken in this group.
- Clinical characteristic can change. Migraine with aura can lose the headache element. Auras can present with any sensory or motor manifestation which in the absence of headache can lead to diagnostic difficulties.
- Migraine has a high co-morbidity with depression, which is already underdiagnosed in this age group.
- All drugs have a higher risk of adverse events.
- Use triptans with caution (see Table 16.2).

Hypnic headache
- A benign and rare disorder of the elderly. See Table 16.3.
- It occurs most frequently in the entire head, but occasionally hemicranially.
- The headache is only during the night and frequently at the same time.
- The pain is moderate to severe and lasts up to 3h.
- Multiple episodes during the night are rare.
- Treatment options include caffeine, lithium carbonate and indometacin.

Table 16.1 The annual prevalence of headache with age—still a common problem

	Troublesome headache (%)		Chronic headache (%) ≥15 days/month	
Age	Women	Men	Women	Men
20–29	11.6	4.4	2.5	0.9
30–39	11.7	5.6	2.5	1.4
40–49	10.9	6.1	3.2	1.8
50–59	10.4	5.9	3.3	2.5
60–69	8.4	4.5	3.2	1.9
70–79	6.3	4.3	2.4	2.4
80+	6.1	4.6	2.3	2.6
All ages	10.1	5.3	2.8	1.9

Table 16.2 Problems with the use of triptans

- Triptans are unlicensed for those over 65 years
- This is because industry was reluctant to undertake licensing studies due to the small market and increased background prevalence of ischaemic heart disease
- Providing there are no cardiovascular system contraindications, benefits may be greater than potential risks.
- For medico-legal purposes, an ECG may be advisable

Table 16.3 IHS diagnostic criteria for hypnic headache

A. Dull headache fulfilling criteria B–D
B. Develops only during sleep and awakens patient
C. At least two of the following characteristics:
   1. Occurs >15 times a month
   2. Lasts more than 15min after waking
   3. First occurs after the age of 50
D. No autonomic symptoms and no more than one of nausea, photophobia or photophobia
E. Not attributed to any other disorder

Important secondary headaches in the elderly

Some important headaches in the elderly are shown in Table 16.4. Of note:

- Temporal arteritis (see Chapter 13)
  - Always consider in a patient presenting with a headache over the age of 50.
  - Can mimic the features of other primary headaches although headache gradually worsens with time.
  - Features can include jaw claudication and constitutional symptoms.
  - A raised ESR is a most important indicator but can be normal in some cases.
- Headache associated with brain tumour
  - The incidence of primary brain tumours is 6–10/100 000 population/year of which 70% will present above the age of 50.
  - Although most patients will complain of headaches in the final stages of their disease, incidence at the time of diagnosis is between 23 and 56%.
  - Headache as an isolated presentation is much lower: 2–16%.
  - A new headache presentation over the age of 50 should always be treated with suspicion.

Table 16.4 Important causes of headache in the elderly

- Space-occupying lesions
- Temporal arteritis
- Trigeminal neuralgia
- Post-herpetic neuralgia
- Systemic disease, e.g. anaemia, hypocalcaemia, hyponatremia, renal failure
- Cerebral vascular disease (thrombotic and embolic stroke—headache in 20–40%, intracerebral haemorrhage—headache in 80%, SAH—headache in 95%)
- Parkinson disease (possibly due to muscle rigidity)
- Hypoxia or hypercapnia
- Cervical spondylosis
- Paget's disease

Chapter 17

Facial pain

Introduction

Facial pain is common in primary care and hospital-based practice, and a multidisciplinary approach involving the GP, neurologist and otolaryngologist is often required.

Facial pain associated with rhinosinusitis

Clinical features

- Sinusitis is defined as inflammation of the mucous membranes of the nasal cavity and paranasal sinuses, fluids within these cavities and/or the underlying bone. Diagnosed by the presence of two or more of:
  - Facial pain
  - Nasal obstruction
  - Nasal discharge (purulent) or discoloured post-nasal drainage
  - Altered sense of smell (hyposmia/anosmia).
- Character of pain:
  - Dull ache, pressure or heaviness.
  - Distributed over the nasal bridge, maxillary, orbital and frontal areas.
  - Worse during an upper respiratory tract infection and when stooping.
  - Pain associated with a frontal sinusitis is typically worse in the morning (vacuum headache).
  - Pain associated with sphenoiditis is usually described as deep-seated and referred to the vertex.
  - Ethmoiditis usually results in pain between the eyes.
- Patients with rhinosinusitis may also suffer from headaches, halitosis, fatigue, dental pain, cough or ear pressure/fullness.
- Chronic rhinosinusitis is sinusitis lasting >12 weeks.

Pathophysiology

- Facial pain can be caused by a deviated nasal septum impacted against the lateral nasal wall or a rhinitic mucosa with turbinate hypertrophy in contact with the septal mucosas.
- The aetiology of this facial pain is uncertain. Theories include local release of substance P and referred pain.
- The afferent fibres from pain receptors in the nasal mucosa terminate in the same group of sensory neurons in the sensory nucleus of the trigeminal nerve as fibres innervating cutaneous receptors, located at several peripheral segmental dermatomes of the ophthalmic and maxillary divisions of the trigeminal nerve. These two common pathways converge along the same final neurons to a common area of the cortex.
- The brain cannot distinguish the original peripheral source of the pain impulses and they may be misinterpreted as coming from other skin areas, such as the temple, the zygoma or the forehead.

Table 17.1 Diagnostic approach to patients with facial pain

- History
  - Age of onset
  - Frequency and timing of attacks
  - Distribution of the pain
  - Character, aggravating and alleviating factors
  - Response to treatment
  - Associated symptoms such as nausea, vomiting, visual disturbance
  - History of head injuries, intracranial infections, surgery, medical and psychiatric illnesses
  - Current medications including over-the-counter analgesics.
- Examination
  - The extent of the physical examination is determined by the history.
  - All patients require a complete head and neck and neurological examinations. This includes evaluation of the cranial nerves, ophthalmic examination with fundoscopy, evaluation of the temporo-mandibular joints for jaw opening, tenderness/creptius, tenderness over muscles of mastication/occipital area and dental examination.
  - An ear, nose and throat examination can be carried out adequately using an otoscope, looking for evidence of pus or polyps in nasal cavities.
- Investigations
  - Investigations to exclude a systemic illness are requested according to the findings in the history and clinical examination.
  - CT of the head and sinuses and an MRI scan of the brain are requested in the presence of unexplained findings or where a definite diagnosis has not been made.

The pain may be perceived also from other end-organs innervated by terminal branches within the trigeminal system, such as dura, intracranial and scalp vessels or the eye

Examination
- In patients with anterior ethmoiditis, frontal and maxillary sinusitis, purulent discharge and oedematous mucosa are often seen in the region of the middle meatus (lateral to the middle turbinate).
- In patients with sphenoiditis, the pus is often found medial to the middle turbinate as it arises from the spheno-ethmoidal recess.
- In chronic rhinosinusitis, examination may reveal the presence of nasal polyps.

Investigations
- The Royal College of Radiologists has recommended that plain X-rays are not used for the diagnosis of rhinosinusitis.
- In selected patients where the signs of rhinosinusitis are not evident clinically, a high resolution CT scan of the sinuses (coronal cuts) is used to confirm the diagnosis.
  - There is a poor correlation between the findings on the CT scan and the localization of the facial pain by the patient.
  - A CT scan is also required to exclude malignancy in patients with atypical symptoms, e.g. unilateral purulent nasal discharge that may be blood stained, and in the presence of a unilateral nasal polyp or mass.

Treatment
- Acute rhinosinusitis >5 days, a broad-spectrum antibiotic such as amoxicillin or co-amoxiclav prescribed for 10 days. In addition, a topical steroid nasal spray should be used.
- For chronic rhinosinusitis, a broad-spectrum antibiotic should be given for longer periods (6–12 weeks) together with a steroid nasal spray for 12 weeks.
- Patients who fail the above treatment should be referred to an otolaryngologist for consideration of endoscopic sinus surgery.
- Sinonasal tumours constitute a wide variety of benign and malignant neoplasms.
  - Benign tumours include inverted papillomas, osteomas, giant cell granulomas and neurogenic tumours.
  - Malignant tumours are rare and represent <1% of all malignancies. Squamous cell carcinoma is the most common pathology (80%).
  - Other tumours include adenocarcinoma, adenoid cystic carcinoma and olfactory neuroblastoma.
- Pain is usually a result of infiltration of the sensory branches of the trigeminal nerve or a secondary sinusitis.

Primary headaches
Tension-type headaches, migraine and cluster can cause facial pain.

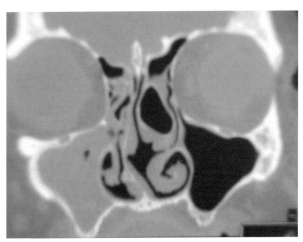

Fig. 17.1 Coronal CT scan in a patient with chronic maxillary sinusitis and right facial pain.

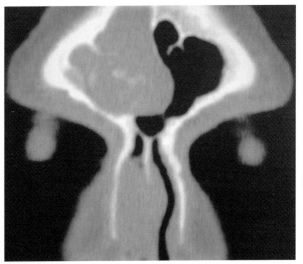

Fig. 17.2 CT scan of a patient with right frontal pain and right frontal sinusitis.

Facial neuralgias

- Trigeminal neuralgia. The most common of the facial neuralgias. Invariably presents over the age of 50 and more common in women (see Table 17.2).
- Mid-facial segment pain
  - Facial neuralgia that has the characteristics of TTH except it affects the mid-face.
  - Described as a feeling of pressure, although some patients might feel that their nose is blocked when they have no nasal airway obstruction.
  - Symmetric and can involve the root, under the bridge or on either side of the nose, the peri or retro-orbital regions, or across the cheeks.
  - There might be hyperaesthesia of the skin and soft tissues over the affected area.
  - Nasal endoscopy and CT scans are typically normal.
  - Treatment is low-dose amitriptyline, but noticeable improvement might require up to 6 weeks of treatment.
- Other rare neuralgias can occur which include:
  - Glossopharyngeal neuralgia—deep stabbing pain in one side of the throat. This can extend into the ear.
  - Geniculate neuralgia—this is a rare neuralgia in the distribution of the nervous intermedius; the somatic sensory branch of cranial nerve VII causes intermittent stabbing pain in the ear.

Post-herpetic neuralgia

- Occurs in patients with a history of herpes zoster infection of one of the branches of the trigeminal nerve.
- The pain persists for 1–6 months after the acute infection.
- No sex difference, but more common and incapacitating with age.
- Pain most commonly affects the distribution of the ophthalmic branch of the trigeminal nerve.
  - A constant burning or aching
  - An episodic, stabbing pain.
  - Both may occur spontaneously and may be aggravated by various stimuli.
- There is hypoaesthesia along the distribution of one of the branches of the trigeminal nerve.
- The early use of antiviral agents such as aciclovir in patients with acute herpes zoster infections may minimize the occurrence of post-herpetic neuralgia.
- TCAs are helpful.

Table 17.2 Features of trigeminal neuralgia

- The course may fluctuate over many years with periods of remission.
- Pain is unilateral.
- Described as stabbing or burning pain.
- Pain restricted to one of the 3 main sensory branches of the trigeminal nerve.
- Physical examination is typically normal.
- Mild light touch or pin perception loss has been described in the nasolabial fold on the same side of the pain.
- Electrophysiological investigations show sensory abnormalities in modalities of the trigeminal nerve that corresponded to the triggered zone.
- Significant sensory loss suggests that the pain syndrome is secondary to another pathology. An MRI should be performed to rule out intracranial pathology mainly in the posterior cranial fossa. This includes lesions compressing the trigeminal nerve roots, e.g. mass lesions, vascular ectasia and malformations.
- The standard drug of choice is carbamazepine, but gabapentin can also be used.
- Invasive interventions include microvascular decompression, neurectomies, radiofrequency, thermal ablation and radiosurgery.

Table 17.3 Features of dental pain

- Pain from dental pulp
  - Can present with mid-face or temporal pain
  - Dental abscess can present similarly
- Atypical odontalgia
  - Acute pain indistinguishable from pulp pain but often more disabling
  - Only transiently relieved by tooth removal
  - Probably neuropathic

Temporomandibular disorder

- Temporomandibular disorder (TMD) is pain and/or dysfunction of the masticatory apparatus.
- TMD comprises 2 syndromes which can be present at the same time, making diagnosis and treatment more challenging:
  - Muscle-related TMD (myogenous), sometimes called TMD secondary to myofacial pain
  - Joint-related (arthrogenous). TMD secondary to true articular disease.
- Can be a history of trauma, e.g. procedures that necessitate jaw extension such as tonsillectomy, endoscopy and molar extraction.
- The pain usually arises in the ear and is referred to the temple, cheek or neck.
- Associated symptoms include a crepitus or a click and pain on movement of the joint.
- Limited opening or locking of the jaw may occur.
- Examination often demonstrates
  - Tenderness of the condyle
  - Compromised mandibular movements, temporomandibular
  - Joint sounds and dental changes, such as incisal edge wear and excessive overbite.
- An MRI scan of the temporomandibular joints is the investigation of choice. Internal derangement (i.e. disk displacement or deformation) and degenerative joint disease are the most common findings.
- Treatment
  - Conservative treatment includes use of NSAIDs, soft diet, avoidance of excessive gum chewing, jaw clenching and teeth grinding.
  - The use of jaw splints (bite plates) may be useful.
  - Intratricular steroids/local anaesthetic injections and arthroscopic surgery are used in severe cases refractory to treatment.

Chronic idiopathic facial pain (atypical facial pain)

- A syndrome encompassing a wide group of facial pain presentations that do not fit any of the above diagnoses. The exact cause remains unclear.
- Described as burning, aching or cramping.
- On one side of the face, often in the region of the trigeminal nerve and can extend into the upper neck or back of the scalp.
- Continuous with few remissions, but is less intense that the pain associated with trigeminal neuralgia.
- Does not usually respond to standard analgesia, antibiotics or steroid nasal sprays. Pain will usually persist despite numerous treatments and interventions by otolaryngologist, physicians and dentists.
- The diagnosis of atypical facial pain is one of exclusion. A meticulous neurological, dental and otolaryngological evaluation is necessary to exclude other causes of facial pain. A CT scan of the brain and sinuses may help exclude other aetiologies.
- Medical treatment is the preferred option and includes amitriptyline.

Alternative approaches where evidence is awaited or contested

Psychology in headache management

The current understanding of headache sits within a biopsychosocial framework. Headache sufferers and in particular migraineurs have higher levels of anxiety and depression than and may demonstrate different personality and behavioural characteristics from those without headache. However, the mechanism of these factors is complex and likely to be bidirectional.

While recognizing that there are few strictly psychogenic headaches, psychology intervention can modulate emotional factors, offer strategies that can help the patient cope with their pain more effectively and provide an important therapeutic input to the management of headache based on a team approach.

Psychological testing

- Can contribute to understanding psychological co-morbidity and coping strategies.
- Can be helpful where:
  - There is a history of psychological co-morbidity.
  - Complex headache history.
  - Multiple treatment failures.
  - Difficulties with obtaining a headache history.
  - When considering treatments that may have psychological side effects, e.g. β-blockers in patients who may be depressed.
  - When there are problems with compliance.
  - When appropriate medication does not lead to anticipated improvement.
- Among the tests that have gained credence in the headache field are the MMPI-2, MBHI and BDI-I (see Table 18.1).

Psychological treatment

Cognitive-behavioural therapy (CBT)

- An approach that emphasizes the present and that we have the ability to overcome difficulties and gain greater control over our emotions and our functioning through our ability to think.
- Emotional distress is maintained through passive acceptance of situations perceived as being beyond our control and/or assuming the worst through 'catastrophizing'—the cognitive process through which an objectively unpleasant current situation is given a tragic and permanent quality.
- Catastrophizing is maintained through an irrational belief system.
  - If unchallenged it becomes an accepted part of the individual's personality.
  - Resists change because of the expectation that the effort involved won't lead to a helpful outcome.
  - Plants the seeds of medication overuse, noncompliance, and depression.

Table 18.1 Psychological tests for use with headache patients

- MMPI-2 (Minnesota Multiphasic Personality Inventory 2)
  - Lengthy inventory taking ~1h
  - Most widely researched personality test providing a number of scales across clinical and psychological elements
- MBMD (Million Behavioral Medicine Diagnostic)
  - Can be completed in <30min
  - Specifically designed for medical settings
  - Reported in more medical terms than the mental health terms favoured by MMPI-2
  - Not as widely researched in headache populations but, in view of relative brevity and health-related orientation, holds future promise
- BDI-11 (Beck Depression Inventory-11)
  - A brief self-report instrument that is a measure of mood
  - Can be prone to false negatives when patients are guarded or uncomfortable about disclosing their distress

- CBT provides the patient with skills to challenge erroneous beliefs and to implement behaviours to change unhappy circumstances.
- Patients become partners in their treatment and reduce the centrality of pain in their lives.
- CBT can be particularly effective when belief systems have been compromised because of feelings of:
  - Unfairness ('I didn't do anything to cause my headaches')
  - Failure ('I've done everything that the doctors have asked of me, and I can't get rid of my headaches')
  - Negative self-attributes ('Other people get headaches; they take a pill and it goes away. I'm different from everybody else')
  - Catastrophic fantasies ('I'll never get better, and I can't go on living like this,' or 'The fact that my headache continues is evidence of the fact that my disease is so terrible that the doctors have been unable to figure it out).
- Rather than being passive recipients of medications, patients can learn to challenge irrational thinking that can limit quality of life. For example:
  - 'What's the worst thing that can happen if I decide to go out with friends and then get a headache?'
  - 'How do I know that my headache will never improve?'
  - 'Will taking less pain medication have potentially tragic consequences or just be uncomfortable?'
- Once patients begin to acknowledge that their thoughts are not facts, and they are open to question, they can begin to develop alternative ways of thinking, such as:
  - 'Having a headache is no fun, but it doesn't have to permanently limit me.'
  - 'I don't know if I will get a disabling headache, but I will be able to deal with it.'
  - 'The bad stuff has been ruled out, and the doctors continue to treat me, so I obviously might get better'.
- Patients who are able to challenge and overcome erroneous beliefs can learn to implement behaviour plans that can be rewarding in various ways, including reducing medication usage, increasing activity levels, and making headache a less significant part of the self-image.
- The patient's ability to use CBT effectively is enhanced by the physician who has a non-fatalistic attitude about headache and is able to remain a role model of positive thinking even in light of a series of failed treatments.

Psychodynamic treatment
May be indicated if post-traumatic stress or if dissociative features are relevant.

Family therapy
If headache has a function in maintaining the family structure or arises from family dysfunction, family therapy may be the initial treatment of choice.

Biofeedback
- By learning relaxation strategies while monitoring physiological responses, aspects of physiology that are assumed to be involuntary can be controlled (e.g. breathing rate, muscle tension, peripheral skin temperature, EEG and pulse rate.
- There is evidence of beneficial effects of hand warming and reduction of muscle tension in headache control.
- Biofeedback is helpful in addressing the anxiety that is associated with headache.
- Can be used in conjunction with preventative medication.
- Where medication may not be desirable, can be used alone (e.g. pregnant women, children and adolescents, patients who prefer non-pharmacological treatments).
- Biofeedback and all relaxation strategies require practice and commitment.

Acupuncture

Background

- Acupuncture is the placing of a solid needle into the body (piercing the skin) for therapeutic purposes. It was developed in China and dates back to ~2000BC.
- The majority of acupuncture treatment in the UK is provided in private practice by professional (lay) acupuncturists who are due to be statutorily regulated following the recommendations of the House of Lords Science and Technology Report into Complementary Medicine (2000).
- The British Medical Acupuncture Society (www.medical-acupuncture. co.uk) was founded in 1980 and has trained >5000 UK healthcare professionals in acupuncture.
- There are a large number of variables in the technique which makes comparisons difficult. e.g. sites, number of needles, depth of insertion, method of stimulation.

Types of acupuncture

- Acupuncture should usually be given for a minimum of 6–8 sessions before being assumed to be ineffective, starting at weekly or twice-weekly intervals. Most clinical trials in chronic headache have used a protocol consisting of 10–15 sessions at weekly intervals.
- A number of approaches are recognized.

Traditional Chinese acupuncture

- Traditional Chinese concepts describe illness and disease as a disturbance of qi (a form of energy or 'vital force') within the body.
- *Qi* is said to flow along 12 bilateral and 2 midline *meridians* on the body surface on which the acupuncture points are situated. Many of these correspond to points at which small nerve bundles penetrate fascia.
- The diagnosis is often expressed in terms of imbalances between yin and yang; the aim is to re-establish the correct flow of *qi* throughout the meridians. Treatment is often combined with dietary advice and Chinese herbal treatment.

Western medical acupuncture

- The Western style is a contemporary scientific approach, which is principally based on the neurophysiological mechanisms of needling that influence peripheral and central sites.

Trigger point acupuncture

- Trigger points are hypersensitive points in muscle which are exquisitely tender when palpated through overlying skin.
- They were derived empirically by Western physicians in the late 20th century with a correspondence between trigger points and classical acupuncture points
- Pain may be referred to distant sites which may reproduce the symptoms of the patient.

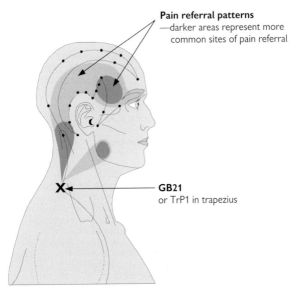

Pain referral patterns
—darker areas represent more
common sites of pain referral

GB21
or TrP1 in trapezius

X←

Fig. 18.1 Pain referral areas from a common trigger point in the upper fibres of trapezius (TrP1) and its overlap with the upper section of the 'Gallbladder' meridian in Traditional Chinese Medicine. Reproduced with permission of the Medical Director, British Acupuncture Society.

- Palpation may elicit a twitch within the band of muscle, and the patient may experience a brief pain.
- Needling of these points even transiently may often produce an impressive reduction of the associated pain.
- A typical trigger point for both cervicogenic headache and migraine is shown in Fig. 18.1. This is also known as 'Gallbladder 21' in traditional Chinese acupuncture, an important point for headache treatment.

Electroacupuncture

- A low intensity (1–12mA) square-wave biphasic current with a frequency of between 2 and 80Hz is applied across pairs of acupuncture needles for up to 30min.
- It is not generally used for headache treatment.

Evidence for acupuncture

- No recent guidelines are available for headache.
- Acupuncture studies in headache have concentrated almost entirely on the prevention of headache rather than its acute treatment.
- A Cochrane Review published in 2001 concluded that 'the existing evidence supports the value of acupuncture for the treatment of idiopathic headaches', but called for further large-scale studies.
- Large, prospective, RCTs are viewed by advocates as showing:
  - Persistent and clinically relevant benefits under real-life conditions and equivalence to drug management (see Fig. 18.2).
  - Similar benefit for 'sham' acupuncture (superficial insertion of needles into non-acupuncture points at both local and distant sites). However, what constitutes valid 'sham' acupuncture is debated.
  - Cost-effectiveness in pragmatic studies
  - The area remains contested. It has been suggested that due to the sham studies there is currently no body of objective evidence to support the routine use of acupuncture in headache.

Safety of acupuncture

- Prospective data collection indicates that acupuncture is extremely safe if delivered by adequately trained practitioners.
- Mild, most frequent adverse events include
  - Momentary pain during needle insertion.
  - Minor bruising or bleeding, usually on needle withdrawal (3%)
  - Worsening of existing symptoms (3%), usually transient (24–48h) and sometimes associated with a good overall outcome
  - Drowsiness, relaxation or euphoria (patients should be advised not to drive to their first appointment). Often experienced as pleasurable.
  - Fainting (<1%)—the first session should always be performed with the patient lying down.
- Severe, rare adverse effects:
  - Haemopericardium or pneumothorax—this is avoided by correct technique

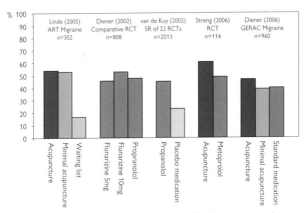

Fig. 18.2 A summary of response rates in recent studies of acupuncture in chronic headache, including direct and indirect comparison with drug treatments. ART = acupuncture randomized trials; RCT = randomized controlled trials; SR = systematic review; GERAC = German acupuncture trials. Reproduced with permission from the Medical Director, British Acupuncture Society.

- Transmission of blood-borne diseases (e.g. hepatitis C)—this is avoided principally by using single-use, sterile, disposable needles.
- Cellulitis or perichondritis—possible with auricular acupuncture, particularly if indwelling studs are used.
- Broken needles (rare with high-quality modern stainless steel needles).

A simple acupuncture protocol for headache

- Those with adequate training could use a formula of 'essential' acupuncture points contained within almost all the clinical trial protocols, consisting of bilateral intramuscular needling at Liver 3, Gallbladder 20 and Gallbladder 21. This is illustrated in Figure 18.3a and b. Gallbladder 20 is the site of occipital nerve injection.
- Needles can be left for 15–20min after assessing immediate response at the first session.
- Continue for 8–10 sessions at weekly intervals and assess overall response using headache diaries.

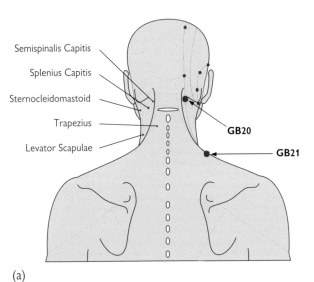

Semispinalis Capitis

Splenius Capitis

Sternocleidomastoid

Trapezius

Levator Scapulae

GB20

GB21

(a)

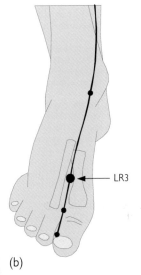

LR3

(b)

Fig. 18.3 A standardized acupuncture protocol for chronic headache.
(a) Gallbladder (GB); (b) liver (LR). Reproduced with permission from the Medical Director, British Acupuncture Society.

Homeopathy

Homeopathy is a therapeutic method using preparations of substances whose effects when administered to healthy people correspond to the manifestations of the disorder (symptoms, clinical signs, pathological states) in the individual patient.

Background

- The principle of homeopathy was expressed by the originator of the method, Dr Samuel Hahnemann (1755–1843) in the latin phrase *similia similibus curentur* (let like be cured by like).
- The fundamental principle of homeopathy is the similia principle.
- He collected as much information as he could about the effect of the pure substance upon people, codifying reports of inadvertent poisonings and performing a large number of tests on volunteers which he termed 'provings'. Here, the participants took the medicine and wrote down all the effects it had on them, physical and emotional.
- The well-known use of extremely dilute medicines is often supposed to be essential, but it is the mode of prescription according to the similia principle which defines homeopathy.
- In the UK, homeopathic hospitals exist within the NHS organization, and GPs are able to prescribe from a list of homeopathic medicines.

Preparation of homeopathic compounds

- Most compounds come from plants, but the list of substances now made into homeopathic remedies (~2500) includes snake venoms, spiders, animal milks and many inorganic salts and other compounds. Anything which has a particular relationship with humankind is a potential homeopathic remedy.
- The job of the homeopathic physician becomes one of teasing out the way an individual patient relates to their world and the detail of how they express their suffering, and analogizing, according to the similia principle, with a substance which has a not dissimilar relationship to the natural world.
- Remedies are often made from preparations of the starting substance which are very dilute indeed. Hahnemann discovered that the good effect of the remedy was maintained while the adverse effects were removed, with dilution critically followed at each step by vigorous shaking ('sucussion').
- Homeopathic remedies are prepared from extracts of the original substances, and these are serially diluted with sucussion of the resulting solution between each step to produce the required strength (or 'potency').
- There are two commonly used scales of dilution. The 'X' or 'D' (decimal) scale dilutes 1 drop in 9 at each step. The 'C' (centesimal) scale dilutes 1 drop in 99 at each step.
- Homeopathic remedies are described by naming the source, then the number of dilution steps and then the scale used, e.g. Sulphur 30C

Table 18.2 Some illustrative cases

Case 1

- 8 year old history of migraine without aura.
- Sent to homeopathic hospital as 'last resort'.
- Characteristics of presentation:
  - Approach to life was straightforward and uncomplicated
  - Had to lie absolutely still in an attack and unable to move eyes
- 30C potency of Bryonia (wild hops)
  - Given for 3 weeks and no recurrence.

Case 2

- Primary exertional headache
- Unable to play sport
- MRI normal
- All conventional treatment ineffective.
- His wife emphasized how irritable and angry the symptoms made him.
- Given nux vomica 30C, 200C, 1000C over 3 days and then 30C twice weekly.
- Headache responded rapidly and gradually returned to normal.

Case 3

- Female with menstrual migraine without aura
- Main concern was the family
- Headache could be exacerbated by warm or stuffy atmospheres and she might often sleep with the window open.
- Pulsatilla (from the wind flower) 30C given daily
- Headache attacks removed

Evidence for homeopathy

- Critics suggest that effects are a function of long consultation times and empathetic listening needed to gain deep understanding of the patients' predicament.
- Benefit has been demonstrated in placebo-controlled trials, but methodology often suffers from lack of rigour.
- Rigorous research has been inhibited by lack of funding and research infrastructure as it has never been supported by the pharmaceutical industry.
- It is claimed that RCTs are not the best way to show the health benefits of homeopathy or of other Complementary and Alternative Medicines

Homeopathy and headache

- There is more 'evidence' for the use of homeopathy in headache than in most other conditions.
- There are at least 4 RCTs of homeopathy in chronic headache (mostly migraine) against placebo. One is very positive, two are equivocal and one is negative.
- Recent prospective, uncontrolled studies which much more closely reflect physicians' and patients' experiences have shown significant improvements in measures of quality of life. For example, of 163 patients studied prospectively at the Bristol homeopathic hospital with a diagnosis of migraine, 53% rated themselves as better and 26% much better after homeopathy.

Table 18.3 Some suggestions that can be prescribed in primary care

To start with, use the 30C potency taken twice weekly.

- Headache coming on since an emotional shock (e.g. witnessing an accident, PTSD, etc.) ACONITE
- Headache starting with a grief (e.g. bereavement) IGNATIA
- PTH (includes stroke or post-surgical) injury especially to skull ARNICA, to neck (e.g. whiplash) NATRUM SULPHURICUM
- To aid medication overuse withdrawal NUX VOMICA (use daily and prn)

Botulinum toxin

Botulinum toxin is used in a wide range of conditions, particularly muscle disorders characterized by excessive muscle contraction such as dystonia and spasticity. William Binder (1992) was the first to report lessening headaches in patients treated for forehead wrinkles. However, its use in primary headache disorders remains controversial.

Mode of action

- Botulinum toxin type A (BoNTA) blocks exocytosis of acetylcholine at the neuromuscular junction.
- BoNTA blocks pain mediators such as substance P and calcitonin gene-related peptide in the peripheral neurons, which may account for its potential effect in pain disorders and headache.

Treatment

There are two treatment approaches for treating headache patients with BoNTA, and both approaches yield similar results:
- The injection at fixed sites in various pericranial muscles (frontalis, temporalis, occipitalis, splenius capitis and trapezius) using 25–100 units of BoNTA.
- Injections at tender points using the same dose.

Evidence base

- All studies confirm that the BoNTA is safe and side effects are minimal.
- Although results have been mixed, the consensus is that there is no benefit in episodic migraine and TTH.
- The results with chronic migraines and chronic TTHs are more promising. The results of large, well controlled studies in these areas are awaited.
- In summary, there is no convincing evidence for use of BoNTA in primary headaches particularly in the prophylaxis of infrequent migraines and TTHs. However, results in patients with more frequent primary headaches indicate a trend towards improvement in the number of headache days and attack frequency.

PFO closure

Background

During foetal development, the foramen ovale allows blood to flow from the right to left atrium, facilitating circulation of oxygenated blood to the foetus. Anatomical closure usually occurs during early childhood, but remains patent maintaining a right-to-left shunt, in 27.6% of the population. 20.3% have a small and 7.3% a large shunt.

Closure of the patent foramen ovale (PFO) using an implantation procedure is used clinically in the treatment of stroke and decompression illness. There may be the potential for treating migraine with aura (MA) by PFO closure .

- There is persuasive evidence of an epidemiological link between MA and the presence of PFOs.
- Observational studies suggest that PFO closure in affected patients leads to the resolution or improvement of MA in the majority of patients.
- The first prospective, randomized and controlled clinical study was negative, and further studies are awaited.
- At the time of writing, there is no good evidence for PFO closure.

Possible mechanism

- Link may be co-morbid not causal.
- PFOs may favour MA attacks in genetically predisposed subjects by allowing vasoactive substances, platelet emboli or paradoxical emboli to bypass the lung filter and trigger the cortical spreading depression of the aura.

Epidemiological studies

These suggest a bidirectional link between PFO and MA, which may have a genetic component. There is no persuasive evidence for a link between PFO and MO.

- The prevalence of migraine is very high in patients with PFO.
  - Right-to-left shunts demonstrate an overall prevalence of migraine of 22–57%, MA of 18–43% and MO of 14–21%. These are all significantly higher than population values.
  - MA increased with the size of the right-to-left shunt, from 4% with small shunts to 25% with medium, and to 53% with large shunts.
- The prevalence of PFO in MA is higher than expected.
  - 41–48% of patients have PFO associated with MA, compared with 16–20% in control subjects without migraine.
  - The prevalence of PFO in patients with MO is similar to that of control patients.
- A genetic study demonstrated autosomal dominant inheritance of PFOs and other atrial shunts, with a genetic linkage to inheritance of MA.

Table 18.4 Key points

- There is a direct epidemiological relationship between MA and the severity of PFO shunts.
- PFO cannot be heard on direct auscultation or identified on routine echocardiography.
- Data from retrospective and open studies indicate that PFO closure may be highly effective in resolving or improving MA attacks.
- Further research is required before PFO closure can be recommended as a treatment for MA.
- The closure devices remain for investigational use at present.

Evidence from clinical studies

- Data are derived from retrospective analyses or prospective open studies that are non-randomized, unblinded and uncontrolled, in highly selected populations.
- PFO closure by transcatheter and surgical procedures has become a commonly used procedure to treat cryptogenic stroke, TIAs and decompression sickness in divers (Table 18.4).
  - Overall, 70–91% of patients report resolution or improvement.
  - Prospective studies demonstrate greater effectiveness than conventional medical treatments in treating migraine.
  - Low adverse event rates were found when closures were conducted by experienced cardiologists.
- Prospective, randomized, controlled clinical studies are required to confirm the effect of PFO closure on migraine.
  - The 'MIST Trial' was designed to provide Grade A evidence on the efficacy of PFO closure for patients with MA.
  - As yet, the MIST Trial has not been published in full.
  - The trial clearly demonstrated an association between MA and the severity of the PFO shunt. The prevalence of large shunts (mostly PFOs) was ~6 times greater in the MA patients than in the general population.
  - Lessons learned from the MIST Trial will be used to aid in the design of future studies of PFO closure for the treatment of MA.
  - Several devices are currently in early clinical development for PFO closure.

Table 18.5 The MIST study

- The MIST Trial was a prospective, randomized, double-blind placebo-controlled study.
- Patients had severe, refractory migraine with aura. Eligible patients had frequent migraine attacks (≥5 days per month) of MA, and had failed on two different preventive medications.
- Transthoracic contrast echocardiography was used to detect the presence of right-to-left shunts (PFOs, atrial septal defects and pulmonary shunts), and for semi-quantitative assessment of their size.
- Patients with moderate-to-large PFOs were randomized to transcatheter closure of the PFO with the STARFlex® Septal Repair Implant or to a sham placebo procedure.
- Placebo control was effected with a sham procedure under anaesthesia, with blinding preserved for patients and physicians.
- Patients were monitored for a 90 day healing period, followed by a 90 day analysis period.
- The primary efficacy end-point compared the incidence of migraine headache in the two groups during the analysis phase and was negative.

The role of the specialist nurse in headache

Introduction

The terms advanced and specialist nurse encompass a wide range of job titles covering many roles, e.g. clinical nurse specialist, nurse practitioner and nurse consultant.

The role of the specialist nurse has developed and expanded rapidly, promoted by several factors:

- The reduction in junior doctors' hours resulted in nurses extending their role to take on tasks previously performed by junior medical staff.
- The United Kingdom Central Council for Nursing (UKCC) formally recognized two levels of nursing practice beyond initial registration and set out guidelines for role expansion and reforms in nurse education.
- The national service frameworks, stringent government targets for health outcomes, were initiated, together with the belief that advanced nursing roles can make a value contribution to meeting these targets.
- Patients demanded greater choice and accessibility.

From a practical perspective, 10 key roles have been established although not all will apply to a single specialty (see Table 19.1).

Professional and educational requirements

- Registration with the Nursing and Midwifery Council
- Advanced certification not compulsory within the specialty but this is recommended
- Master's level of education is required and supported by many NHS Trusts.

Role development

- Role development is a process of skill acquisition and change in focus of practice through experience
- It is influenced by the individual's potential, background experience and the work setting
- Roles are continuously evolving and expanding
- Due to the complexity of the role, the specialist nurse experiences a development process before being able to function with maximum effectiveness (see Table 19.2).

Constraints to role development

- Lack of time. Regular review of the current workload is required to ensure that the quality of the service is maintained and that the number of tasks undertaken is controlled.
- Lack of understanding among colleagues and patients and failure to embrace the newer way of working within an organization.
- Support from medical staff. The role is firmly rooted in nursing and does not strive to be seen as a new generation within the medical profession.
- Administrative tasks should be limited to allow the specialist nurse to improve patient care. This can be done directly through clinical intervention and indirectly by working in collaboration with other

specialists, members of the multidisciplinary team and administrators in the area of consultation, service planning, education and research.

Table 19.1 Ten key roles as defined by the UK Chief Nursing Officer

- Order diagnostic test
- Make and receive referrals
- Admit and discharge patients
- Manage patient caseloads
- Run clinics
- Prescribe medications/treatments
- Carry out resuscitation procedures
- Triage patients
- Take a lead on the way local services are run
- Minor surgery

Table 19.2 Stages of role development

Increasing confidence through individual direct patient care

Direct care and/or planning with other staff for groups of patients

Working with staff to change the nursing care of patients within a clinical speciality

Conducting and participating in research projects

Planning for changes in patient care delivery based on experience and research

Increasing input into higher levels of the healthcare delivery system

Integrating all role components with confidence

Activities undertaken by the headache nurse

Prescribing

Prescribing remains the responsibility of the doctors.

- Independent nurse prescribers may prescribe any licensed medicine except controlled drugs, and supplementary nurse prescribers can prescribe any medicine in the patient's clinical management plan.
- Nurses may also use PGDs (patient group directions).
- A PGD is an agreement signed by a doctor and agreed by a pharmacist that can act as a direction to a nurse to supply and/or administer prescription-only medicines (POMs) to patients using their own assessment of patient need without necessarily referring back to a doctor for an individual prescription. However, the UK list does not currently include most of the frequently used drugs for headache treatment.
- An alternative method that may be used is to have agreed medication dosing regimes with clear guidelines on dose escalation for individual medicines. Here the nurse will not prescribe but will be competent to advise the patient and/or colleague on medication dosing and changes whilst being alert to adverse effects and tolerability issues, and aware of how to optimize the treatment.

Medical practitioner-led outpatient clinics

- Taking a comprehensive headache history.
- Assessing level of disability due to headache.
- Providing advice on lifestyle issues.
- Advising on the use of medication.
- Provision and assessment of diaries that monitor headache.
- Discussion of the case with the headache consultant.

Inpatient care

- Assessing educational and training needs of ward staff that will be caring for this patient group.
- Providing regular education and training for ward staff.
- Ensuring understanding of the use of specific medications for headache treatment.
- Developing drug administration guidelines and care plans for specific treatments.
- Developing plans of care to meet patient needs, e.g. analgesia withdrawal.
- Supporting the clinical team caring for headache patients.
- Assessing the healthcare needs of patients.
- Ensuring the patient understands their plan of care in hospital.
- Monitoring progress and ensuring care is optimized.
- Working with ward staff to minimize, recognize and treat any adverse effects promptly.
- Providing health promotion and advice for patients on coping with their headache.

- Ensuring the patient understands the management plan prior to discharge.
- Clarifying use of medications and dosing regimes.

Telephone role

- Monitoring patient progress at intervals following inpatient treatment.
- Monitoring drug efficacy and side effects.
- Supporting patients with changes in treatment.
- Accessible to provide additional support through telephone contact.
- Any change in medical treatment from the established plan or significant development is discussed with and addressed by the headache consultant.

Organizational activities

- Collaborating with management and clinical team to focus on service delivery and service development issues.
- Working with administration departments to coordinate various aspects of the service that impact on in- and outpatient activity.
- Teaching on nursing courses within the organization.
- Support/education input at the local headache charity.
- Working with other specialist nurses to develop the profile and establish the role nationally.

Conclusion

- The specialist headache nurse's role is a non-traditional one with expanded boundaries.
- Due to the complexity of the role, the nurse experiences a role development process.
- The best preparation for these roles is a combination of having the right experience together with suitable educational background.
- New knowledge in headache and the availability of new treatments have made headache management more effective, but also more complex.
- The specialist nurse can facilitate both inpatient and outpatient care.
- One way of improving a headache service is by regular follow-up by a specialist, and this may be through a telephone or outpatient clinic.
- Access to the headache nurse specialist who has the authority and experience to advise patients on medication and treatment issues is a cost-effective way of providing this patient-focused care.
- A responsive service providing inpatient and outpatient management of complex headache conditions needs to be equipped, coordinated and responsive to patient and service needs. To provide a safe and effective service, the specialist nurse should have advanced training in headache, relevant experience, access to the patient's medical records and clinical support from a specialist consultant in headache.

Chapter 20

The development of headache services

Introduction

Demographic, epidemiological and socio-economic developments are driving demands for improvements in the efficiency and quality of healthcare delivery. These tensions have resulted in a search for ways of re-aligning healthcare organizations, reflecting a broader agenda to modernize and improve public services as a whole.

Current headache care and service development

- The care that headache sufferers receive is generally poor.
- Less than 50% of patients are satisfied with their current treatment.
- 30% of secondary care consultations are for headache, many of which may be inappropriate for this setting.
- Despite having the highest economic impact amongst neurological diseases, headache receives the lowest research priority.
- To date, the primary research focus has been on the epidemiology, pathophysiology and treatment of headache. The development of more effective models of service delivery may offer greater immediate potential to reduce the burden of headache.

The British Association for the Study of Headache model of care

The development of services will depend on the context and history of each country. There is no evidence base of effectiveness or cost-effectiveness of any model of care. In the UK, the model proposed by The British Association for the Study of Headache is:

- GPs provide care for the majority of patients.
- Intermediate care headache centres staffed by GP with a specialist interest should support front-line GPs (see Tables 20.1, 20.2).
- Neurologists in specialist secondary care centres should support these two levels.
- The importance of specialist nurses and other healthcare professionals is recognised.

Developing an evidence base for service development

- The prevailing scientific methods that direct headache research are underpinned by statistical approaches that may have limited utility in the analysis of complex systems such as headache care delivery.
- Broader research approaches drawing on other methodologies such as qualitative research should be used.

- More useful answers may be obtained from the question of what works for who and what circumstances, rather than seeking generalizable solutions to headache care delivery and overlooking the importance of local context.

Table 20.1 What is a GP with a special interest?

- GPs with special interest deliver a clinical service beyond the normal scope of general practice, undertake advanced procedures or develop services.
- They will work as partners in a managed service not under direct supervision, keeping within their competencies.
- They do not offer a full consultant service and will not replace local consultants or interfere with access to consultants by local GPs.

Table 20.2 Some practical advantages claimed for intermediate care

- Increased patient throughput and clinical capacity
- Services more accessible to patients
- Encourages professional development
- May facilitate retention of medical staff by offering a broader range of interests
- Could release resources from secondary care to see more appropriate cases
- May offer care more efficiently

Table 20.3 Some questions to think about when redesigning headache services.

- Is the aim an addition to the services in existence, complementation, substitution, or a combination of all three?
- Is there a danger that it will simply expose unmet need?
- What are the implications for other services that may be affected directly or indirectly? For example, the introduction of a new service may de-stabilize the delivery of secondary care services.
- What is the best increment in service development to undertake and how should the service be configured?
- Are new resources available or is disinvestment required from secondary care? If so, is this a practical option and can the released resources be identified?
- What are the training and governance requirements. (Guidelines have been developed by the Royal College of General Practitioners defining the competencies required and governance arrangements (www.doh.gov. uk/pricare/gp-specialinterest.) Specific guidance has also been developed for headache.

International Headache Society classification of headache

IHS ICHD-II code	WHO ICD-10NA code	Diagnosis [and aetiological ICD-10 code for secondary headache disorders]
1.	[G43]	Migraine
1.1	[G43.0]	Migraine without aura
1.2	[G43.1]	Migraine with aura
1.2.1	[G43.10]	Typical aura with migraine headache
1.2.2	[G43.10]	Typical aura with non-migraine headache
1.2.3	[G43.104]	Typical aura without headache
1.2.4	[G43.105]	Familial hemiplegic migraine (FHM)
1.2.5	[G43.105]	Sporadic hemiplegic migraine
1.2.6	[G43.103]	Basilar-type migraine
1.3	[G43.82]	Childhood periodic syndromes that are commonly precursors of migraine
1.3.1	[G43.82]	Cyclical vomiting
1.3.2	[G43.820]	Abdominal migraine
1.3.3	[G43.821]	Benign paroxysmal vertigo of childhood
1.4	[G43.81]	Retinal migraine
1.5	[G43.3]	Complications of migraine
1.5.1	[G43.3]	Chronic migraine
1.5.2	[G43.2]	Status migrainosus
1.5.3	[G43.3]	Persistent aura without infarction
1.5.4	[G43.3]	Migrainous infarction
1.5.5	[G43.3] + [G40.x or G41.x]*	Migraine-triggered seizures
1.6	[G43.83]	Probable migraine
1.6.1	[G43.83]	Probable migraine without aura
1.6.2	[G43.83]	Probable migraine with aura
1.6.5	[G43.83]	Probable chronic migraine

Continued

IHS ICHD-II code	WHO ICD-10NA code	Diagnosis [and aetiological ICD-10 code for secondary headache disorders]
2.	**[G44.2]**	**Tension-type headache (TTH)**
2.1	[G44.2]	Infrequent episodic tension-type headache
2.1.1	[G44.20]	Infrequent episodic tension-type headache associated with pericranial tenderness
2.1.2	[G44.21]	Infrequent episodic tension-type headache not associated with pericranial tenderness
2.2	[G44.2]	Frequent episodic tension-type headache
2.2.1	[G44.20]	Frequent episodic tension-type headache associated with pericranial tenderness
2.2.2	[G44.21]	Frequent episodic tension-type headache not associated with pericranial tenderness
2.3	[G44.2]	Chronic tension-type headache
2.3.1	[G44.22]	Chronic tension-type headache associated with pericranial tenderness
2.3.2	[G44.23]	Chronic tension-type headache not associated with pericranial tenderness
2.4	[G44.28]	Probable tension-type headache
2.4.1	[G44.28]	Probable infrequent episodic tension-type headache
2.4.2	[G44.28]	Probable frequent episodic tension-type headache
2.4.3	[G44.28]	Probable chronic tension-type headache
3.	**[G44.0]**	**Cluster headache and other trigeminal autonomic cephalalgias**
3.1	[G44.0]	Cluster headache
3.1.1	[G44.01]	Episodic cluster headache
3.1.2	[G44.02]	Chronic cluster headache
3.2	[G44.03]	Paroxysmal hemicrania
3.2.1	[G44.03]	Episodic paroxysmal hemicrania
3.2.2	[G44.03]	Chronic paroxysmal hemicrania (CPH)
3.3	[G44.08]	Short-lasting unilateral neuralgiform headache attacks with conjunctival injection and tearing (SUNCT)
3.4	[G44.08]	Probable trigeminal autonomic cephalalgia
3.4.1	[G44.08]	Probable cluster headache
3.4.2	[G44.08]	Probable paroxysmal hemicrania
3.4.3	[G44.08]	Probable SUNCT
4.	**[G44.80]**	**Other primary headaches**
4.1	[G44.800]	Primary stabbing headache

IHS ICHD-II code	WHO ICD-10NA code	Diagnosis [and aetiological ICD-10 code for secondary headache disorders]
4.2	[G44.803]	Primary cough headache
4.3	[G44.804]	Primary exertional headache
4.4	[G44.805]	Primary headache associated with sexual activity
4.4.1	[G44.805]	Pre-orgasmic headache
4.4.2	[G44.805]	Orgasmic headache
4.5	[G44.80]	Hypnic headache
4.6	[G44.80]	Primary thunderclap headache
4.7	[G44.80]	Hemicrania continua
4.8	[G44.2]	New daily-persistent headache (NDPH)
5.	**[G44.88]**	**Headache attributed to head and/or neck trauma**
5.1	[G44.880]	Acute post-traumatic headache
5.1.1	[G44.880]	Acute post-traumatic headache attributed to moderate or severe head injury [S06]
5.1.2	[G44.880]	Acute post-traumatic headache attributed to mild head injury [S09.9]
5.2	[G44.3]	Chronic post-traumatic headache
5.2.1	[G44.30]	Chronic post-traumatic headache attributed to moderate or severe head injury [S06]
5.2.2	[G44.31]	Chronic post-traumatic headache attributed to mild head injury [S09.9]
5.3	[G44.841]	Acute headache attributed to whiplash injury [S13.4]
5.4	[G44.841]	Chronic headache attributed to whiplash injury [S13.4]
5.5	[G44.88]	Headache attributed to traumatic intracranial haematoma
5.5.1	[G44.88]	Headache attributed to epidural haematoma [S06.4]
5.5.2	[G44.88]	Headache attributed to subdural haematoma [S06.5]
5.6	[G44.88]	Headache attributed to other head and/or neck trauma [S06]
5.6.1	[G44.88]	Acute headache attributed to other head and/or neck trauma [S06]
5.6.2	[G44.88]	Chronic headache attributed to other head and/or neck trauma [S06]
5.7	[G44.88]	Post-craniotomy headache
5.7.1	[G44.880]	Acute post-craniotomy headache
5.7.2	[G44.30]	Chronic post-craniotomy headache

Continued

IHS ICHD-II code	WHO ICD-10NA code	Diagnosis [and aetiological ICD-10 code for secondary headache disorders]
6.	**[G44.81]**	**Headache attributed to cranial or cervical vascular disorder**
6.1	[G44.810]	Headache attributed to ischaemic stroke or transient ischaemic attack
6.1.1	[G44.810]	Headache attributed to ischaemic stroke (cerebral infarction) [I63]
6.1.2	[G44.810]	Headache attributed to transient ischaemic attack (TIA) [G45]
6.2	[G44.810]	Headache attributed to non-traumatic intracranial haemorrhage [I62]
6.2.1	[G44.810]	Headache attributed to intracerebral haemorrhage [I61]
6.2.2	[G44.810]	Headache attributed to subarachnoid haemorrhage (SAH) [I60]
6.3	[G44.811]	Headache attributed to unruptured vascular malformation [Q28]
6.3.1	[G44.811]	Headache attributed to saccular aneurysm [Q28.3]
6.3.2	[G44.811]	Headache attributed to arteriovenous malformation (AVM) [Q28.2]
6.3.3	[G44.811]	Headache attributed to dural arteriovenous fistula [I67.1]
6.3.4	[G44.811]	Headache attributed to cavernous angioma [D18.0]
6.3.5	[G44.811]	Headache attributed to encephalotrigeminal or leptomeningeal angiomatosis (Sturge–Weber syndrome) [Q85.8]
6.4	[G44.812]	Headache attributed to arteritis [M31]
6.4.1	[G44.812]	Headache attributed to giant cell arteritis (GCA) [M31.6]
6.4.2	[G44.812]	Headache attributed to primary central nervous system (CNS) angiitis [I67.7]
6.4.3	[G44.812]	Headache attributed to secondary central nervous system (CNS) angiitis [I68.2]
6.5	[G44.810]	Carotid or vertebral artery pain [I63.0, I63.2, I65.0, I65.2 or I67.0]
6.5.1	[G44.810]	Headache or facial or neck pain attributed to arterial dissection [I67.0]
6.5.2	[G44.814]	Post-endarterectomy headache [I97.8]
6.5.3	[G44.810]	Carotid angioplasty headache
6.5.4	[G44.810]	Headache attributed to intracranial endovascular procedures

IHS ICHD-II code	WHO ICD-10NA code	Diagnosis [and aetiological ICD-10 code for secondary headache disorders]
6.5.5	[G44.810]	Angiography headache
6.6	[G44.810]	Headache attributed to cerebral venous thrombosis (CVT) [I63.6]
6.7	[G44.81]	Headache attributed to other intracranial vascular disorder
6.7.1	[G44.81]	Cerebral autosomal dominant arteriopathy with subcortical infarcts and leukoencephalopathy (CADASIL) [I67.8]
6.7.2	[G44.81]	Mitochondrial encephalopathy, lactic acidosis and stroke-like episodes (MELAS) [G31.81]
6.7.3	[G44.81]	Headache attributed to benign angiopathy of the central nervous system [I99]
6.7.4	[G44.81]	Headache attributed to pituitary apoplexy [E23.6]
7.	**[G44.82]**	**Headache attributed to non-vascular intracranial disorder**
7.1	[G44.820]	Headache attributed to high cerebrospinal fluid pressure
7.1.1	[G44.820]	Headache attributed to idiopathic intracranial hypertension (IIH) [G93.2]
7.1.2	[G44.820]	Headache attributed to intracranial hypertension secondary to metabolic, toxic or hormonal causes
7.1.3	[G44.820]	Headache attributed to intracranial hypertension secondary to hydrocephalus [G91.8]
7.2	[G44.820]	Headache attributed to low cerebrospinal fluid pressure
7.2.1	[G44.820]	Post-dural puncture headache [G97.0]
7.2.2	[G44.820]	CSF fistula headache [G96.0]
7.2.3	[G44.820]	Headache attributed to spontaneous (or idiopathic) low CSF pressure
7.3	[G44.82]	Headache attributed to non-infectious inflammatory disease
7.3.1	[G44.823]	Headache attributed to neurosarcoidosis [D86.8]
7.3.2	[G44.823]	Headache attributed to aseptic (non-infectious) meningitis [code to specify aetiology]
7.3.3	[G44.823]	Headache attributed to other non-infectious inflammatory disease [code to specify aetiology]

Continued

IHS ICHD-II code	WHO ICD-10NA code	Diagnosis [and aetiological ICD-10 code for secondary headache disorders]
7.3.4	[G44.82]	Headache attributed to lymphocytic hypophysitis [E23.6]
7.4	[G44.822]	Headache attributed to intracranial neoplasm [C00–D48]
7.4.1	[G44.822]	Headache attributed to increased intracranial pressure or hydrocephalus caused by neoplasm [code to specify neoplasm]
7.4.2	[G44.822]	Headache attributed directly to neoplasm [code to specify neoplasm]
7.4.3	[G44.822]	Headache attributed to carcinomatous meningitis [C79.3]
7.4.4	[G44.822]	Headache attributed to hypothalamic or pituitary hyper- or hyposecretion [E23.0]
7.5	[G44.824]	Headache attributed to intrathecal injection [G97.8]
7.6	[G44.82]	Headache attributed to epileptic seizure [G40.x or G41.x to specify seizure type]
7.6.1	[G44.82]	Hemicrania epileptica [G40.x or G41.x to specify seizure type]
7.6.2	[G44.82]	Post-seizure headache [G40.x or G41.x to specify seizure type]
7.7	[G44.82]	Headache attributed to Chiari malformation type I (CM1) [Q07.0]
7.8	[G44.82]	Syndrome of transient headache and neurological deficits with cerebrospinal fluid lymphocytosis (HaNDL)
7.9	[G44.82]	Headache attributed to other non-vascular intracranial disorder
8.	**[G44.4 or G44.83]**	**Headache attributed to a substance or its withdrawal**
8.1	[G44.40]	Headache induced by acute substance use or exposure
8.1.1	[G44.400]	Nitric oxide (NO) donor-induced headache [X44]
8.1.1.1	[G44.400]	Immediate NO donor-induced headache [X44]
8.1.1.2	[G44.400]	Delayed NO donor-induced headache [X44]
8.1.2	[G44.40]	Phosphodiesterase (PDE) inhibitor-induced headache [X44]
8.1.3	[G44.402]	Carbon monoxide-induced headache [X47]
8.1.4	[G44.83]	Alcohol-induced headache [F10]
8.1.4.1	[G44.83]	Immediate alcohol-induced headache [F10]

IHS ICHD-II code	WHO ICD-10NA code	Diagnosis [and aetiological ICD-10 code for secondary headache disorders]
8.1.4.2	[G44.83]	Delayed alcohol-induced headache [F10]
8.1.5	[G44.4]	Headache induced by food components and additives
8.1.5.1	[G44.401]	Monosodium glutamate-induced headache [X44]
8.1.6	[G44.83]	Cocaine-induced headache [F14]
8.1.7	[G44.83]	Cannabis-induced headache [F12]
8.1.8	[G44.40]	Histamine-induced headache [X44]
8.1.8.1	[G44.40]	Immediate histamine-induced headache [X44]
8.1.8.2	[G44.40]	Delayed histamine-induced headache [X44]
8.1.9	[G44.40]	Calcitonin gene-related peptide (CGRP)-induced headache [X44]
8.1.9.1	[G44.40]	Immediate CGRP-induced headache [X44]
8.1.9.2	[G44.40]	Delayed CGRP-induced headache [X44]
8.1.10	[G44.41]	Headache as an acute adverse event attributed to medication used for other indications [code to specify substance]
8.1.11	[G44.4 or G44.83]	Headache attributed to other acute substance use or exposure [code to specify substance]
8.2	[G44.41 or G44.83]	Medication overuse headache (MOH)
8.2.1	[G44.411]	Ergotamine overuse headache [Y52.5]
8.2.2	[G44.41]	Triptan overuse headache
8.2.3	[G44.410]	Analgesic overuse headache [F55.2]
8.2.4	[G44.83]	Opioid overuse headache [F11.2]
8.2.5	[G44.410]	Combination analgesic overuse headache [F55.2]
8.2.6	[G44.41 ± G44.83]	Medication overuse headache attributed to combination of acute medications
8.2.7	[G44.410]	Headache attributed to other medication overuse [code to specify substance]
8.2.8	[G44.41 or G44.83]	Probable medication overuse headache [code to specify substance]
	[G44.4]	Headache as an adverse event attributed to chronic medication [code to specify substance]
	[G44.418]	Exogenous hormone-induced headache [Y42.4]
8.3	[G44.4]	Headache as an adverse event attributed to chronic medication [code to specify substance]
8.3.1	[G44.418]	Exogenous hormone-induced headache [Y42.4]

Continued

IHS ICHD-II code	WHO ICD-10NA code	Diagnosis [and aetiological ICD-10 code for secondary headache disorders]
8.4	[G44.83]	Headache attributed to substance withdrawal
8.4.1	[G44.83]	Caffeine withdrawal headache [F15.3]
8.4.2	[G44.83]	Opioid withdrawal headache [F11.3]
8.4.3	[G44.83]	Oestrogen withdrawal headache [Y42.4]
8.4.4	[G44.83]	Headache attributed to withdrawal from chronic use of other substances [code to specify substance]
9.		**Headache attributed to infection**
9.1	[G44.821]	Headache attributed to intracranial infection [G00–G09]
9.1.1	[G44.821]	Headache attributed to bacterial meningitis [G00.9]
9.1.2	[G44.821]	Headache attributed to lymphocytic meningitis [G03.9]
9.1.3	[G44.821]	Headache attributed to encephalitis [G04.9]
9.1.4	[G44.821]	Headache attributed to brain abscess [G06.0]
9.1.5	[G44.821]	Headache attributed to subdural empyema [G06.2]
9.2	[G44.881]	Headache attributed to systemic infection [A00–B97]
9.2.1	[G44.881]	Headache attributed to systemic bacterial infection [code to specify aetiology]
9.2.2	[G44.881]	Headache attributed to systemic viral infection [code to specify aetiology]
9.2.3	[G44.881]	Headache attributed to other systemic infection [code to specify aetiology]
9.3	[G44.821]	Headache attributed to HIV/AIDS [B22]
9.4	[G44.821 or G44.881]	Chronic post-infection headache [code to specify aetiology]
9.4.1	[G44.821]	Chronic post-bacterial meningitis headache [G00.9]
10.	**[G44.882]**	**Headache attributed to disorder of homeostasis**
10.1	[G44.882]	Headache attributed to hypoxia and/or hypercapnia
10.1.1	[G44.882]	High-altitude headache [W94]
10.1.2	[G44.882]	Diving headache
10.1.3	[G44.882]	Sleep apnoea headache [G47.3]
10.2	[G44.882]	Dialysis headache [Y84.1]
10.3	[G44.813]	Headache attributed to arterial hypertension [I10]

IHS ICHD-II code	WHO ICD-10NA code	Diagnosis [and aetiological ICD-10 code for secondary headache disorders]
10.3.1	[G44.813]	Headache attributed to phaeochromocytoma [D35.0 (benign) or C74.1 (malignant)]
10.3.2	[G44.813]	Headache attributed to hypertensive crisis without hypertensive encephalopathy [I10]
10.3.3	[G44.813]	Headache attributed to hypertensive encephalopathy [I67.4]
10.3.4	[G44.813]	Headache attributed to pre-eclampsia [O13–O14]
10.3.5	[G44.813]	Headache attributed to eclampsia [O15]
10.3.6	[G44.813]	Headache attributed to acute pressor response to an exogenous agent [code to specify aetiology]
10.4	[G44.882]	Headache attributed to hypothyroidism [E03.9]
10.5	[G44.882]	Headache attributed to fasting [T73.0]
10.6	[G44.882]	Cardiac cephalalgia [code to specify aetiology]
10.7	[G44.882]	Headache attributed to other disorders of homeostasis [code to specify aetiology]
11.	**[G44.84]**	**Headache or facial pain attributed to disorder of cranium, neck, eyes, ears, nose, sinuses, teeth, mouth or other facial or cranial structures**
11.1	[G44.840]	Headache attributed to disorder of cranial bone [M80–M89.8]
11.2	[G44.841]	Headache attributed to disorder of neck [M99]
11.2.1	[G44.841]	Cervicogenic headache [M99]
11.2.2	[G44.842]	Headache attributed to retropharyngeal tendonitis [M79.8]
11.2.3	[G44.841]	Headache attributed to craniocervical dystonia [G24]
11.3	[G44.843]	Headache attributed to disorder of eyes
11.3.1	[G44.843]	Headache attributed to acute glaucoma [H40]
11.3.2	[G44.843]	Headache attributed to refractive errors [H52]
11.3.3	[G44.843]	Headache attributed to heterophoria or heterotropia (latent or manifest squint) [H50.3–H50.5]
11.3.4	[G44.843]	Headache attributed to ocular inflammatory disorder [code to specify aetiology]
11.4	[G44.844]	Headache attributed to disorder of ears [H60–H95]
11.5	[G44.845]	Headache attributed to rhinosinusitis [J01]

Continued

IHS ICHD-II code	WHO ICD-10NA code	Diagnosis [and aetiological ICD-10 code for secondary headache disorders]
11.6	[G44.846]	Headache attributed to disorder of teeth, jaws or related structures [K00–K14]
11.7	[G44.846]	Headache or facial pain attributed to temporomandibular joint (TMJ) disorder [K07.6]
11.8	[G44.84]	Headache attributed to other disorder of cranium, neck, eyes, ears, nose, sinuses, teeth, mouth or other facial or cervical structures [code to specify aetiology]
12.	**[R51]**	**Headache attributed to psychiatric disorder**
12.1	[R51]	Headache attributed to somatisation disorder [F45.0]
12.2	[R51]	Headache attributed to psychotic disorder [code to specify aetiology]
13.	**[G44.847, G44.848 or G44.85]**	**Cranial neuralgias and central causes of facial pain**
13.1	[G44.847]	Trigeminal neuralgia
13.1.1	[G44.847]	Classical trigeminal neuralgia [G50.00]
13.1.2	[G44.847]	Symptomatic trigeminal neuralgia [G53.80] + [code to specify aetiology]
13.2	[G44.847]	Glossopharyngeal neuralgia
13.2.1	[G44.847]	Classical glossopharyngeal neuralgia [G52.10]
13.2.2	[G44.847]	Symptomatic glossopharyngeal neuralgia [G53.830] + [code to specify aetiology]
13.3	[G44.847]	Nervus intermedius neuralgia [G51.80]
13.4	[G44.847]	Superior laryngeal neuralgia [G52.20]
13.5	[G44.847]	Nasociliary neuralgia [G52.80]
13.6	[G44.847]	Supraorbital neuralgia [G52.80]
13.7	[G44.847]	Other terminal branch neuralgias [G52.80]
13.8	[G44.847]	Occipital neuralgia [G52.80]
13.9	[G44.851]	Neck–tongue syndrome
13.10	[G44.801]	External compression headache
13.11	[G44.802]	Cold-stimulus headache
13.11.1	[G44.8020]	Headache attributed to external application of a cold stimulus
13.11.2	[G44.8021]	Headache attributed to ingestion or inhalation of a cold stimulus
13.12	[G44.848]	Constant pain caused by compression, irritation or distortion of cranial nerves or upper cervical roots by structural lesions [G53.8] + [code to specify aetiology]

IHS ICHD-II code	WHO ICD-10NA code	Diagnosis [and aetiological ICD-10 code for secondary headache disorders]
13.13	[G44.848]	Optic neuritis [H46]
13.14	[G44.848]	Ocular diabetic neuropathy [E10–E14]
13.15	[G44.881 or G44.847]	Head or facial pain attributed to herpes zoster
13.15.1	[G44.881]	Head or facial pain attributed to acute herpes zoster [B02.2]
13.15.2	[G44.847]	Post-herpetic neuralgia [B02.2]
13.16	[G44.850]	Tolosa–Hunt syndrome
13.17	[G43.80]	Ophthalmoplegic 'migraine'
13.18	[G44.810 or G44.847]	Central causes of facial pain
13.18.1	[G44.847]	Anaesthesia dolorosa [G52.800] + [code to specify aetiology]
13.18.2	[G44.810]	Central post-stroke pain [G46.21]
13.18.3	[G44.847]	Facial pain attributed to multiple sclerosis [G35]
13.18.4	[G44.847]	Persistent idiopathic facial pain [G50.1]
13.18.5	[G44.847]	Burning mouth syndrome [code to specify aetiology]
13.19	[G44.847]	Other cranial neuralgia or other centrally mediated facial pain [code to specify aetiology]
14.	**[R51]**	**Other headache, cranial neuralgia, central or primary facial pain**
14.1	[R51]	Headache not elsewhere classified
14.2	[R51]	Headache unspecified

*The additional code specifies the type of seizure.

(Reproduced with permission)

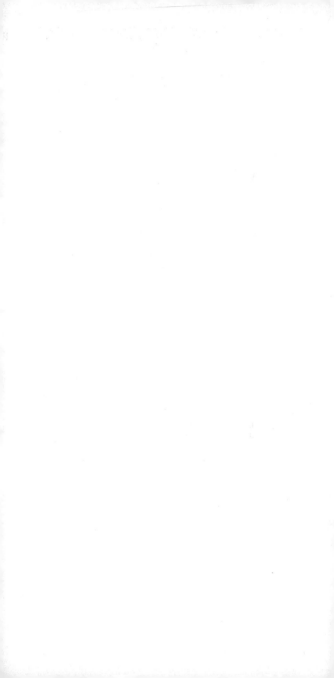

Headache impact questionnaires

Migraine Impact Disability Assessment Score (MIDAS)

1. On how many days did you miss work or school because of your headaches?

   ....

2. How many days was your productivity at work or school reduced by half or more because of your headaches (do not include days you counted in question 1 where you missed work or school)?

   ....

3. On how many days did you not do household work because of your headaches?

   ....

4. How many days was your productivity in household work reduced by half or more because of your headaches (Do not include days you counted in question 3 where you did not do household work)?

   ....

5. On how many days did you miss family, social or leisure activities because of your headaches?

   ....

Scores

0–5 minimal impact
6–10 mild impact
11–20 moderate impact
21+ severe impact

(Reproduced with permission)

Headache Impact Test (HIT)

HIT-6™
(VERSION 1.1)

This questionnaire was designed to help you describe and communicate the way you feel and what you cannot do because of headaches.

To complete, please circle one answer for each question.

HEADACHE

IMPACT TEST™

1 When you have headaches, how often is the pain severe?

| Never | Rarely | Sometimes | Very Often | Always |

2 How often do headaches limit your ability to do usual daily activities including household work, work, school, or social activities?

| Never | Rarely | Sometimes | Very Often | Always |

3 When you have a headache, how often do you wish you could lie down?

| Never | Rarely | Sometimes | Very Often | Always |

4 In the past 4 weeks, how often have you felt too tired to do work or daily activities because of your headaches?

| Never | Rarely | Sometimes | Very Often | Always |

5 In the past 4 weeks, how often have you felt fed up or irritated because of your headaches?

| Never | Rarely | Sometimes | Very Often | Always |

6 In the past 4 weeks, how often did headaches limit your ability to concentrate on work or daily activities?

| Never | Rarely | Sometimes | Very Often | Always |

▽ + ▽ + ▽ + ▽ + ▽

| COLUMN 1 | COLUMN 2 | COLUMN 3 | COLUMN 4 | COLUMN 5 |
| (6 points each) | (8 points each) | (10 points each) | (11 points each) | (13 points each) |

To score, add points for answers in each column.

Please share your HIT-6 results with your doctor.

Total Score

Higher scores indicate greater impact on your life.

Score range is 36–78.

HIT-6™ US (English) Version 1.1
©2000, 2001 QualityMetric, Inc. and GlaxoSmithKline Group of Companies

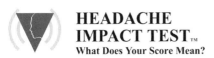

HEADACHE
IMPACT TEST™
What Does Your Score Mean?

▼ **If You Scored 60 or More**

Your headaches are having a very severe impact on your life. You may be experiencing disabling pain and other symptoms that are more severe than those of other headache sufferers. Don't let your headaches stop you from enjoying the important things in your life, like family, work, school or social activities.

Make an appointment **today** to discuss your HIT-6 results and your headaches with your doctor.

▼ **If You Scored 56 – 59**

Your headaches are having a substantial impact on your life. As a result you may be experiencing severe pain and other symptoms, causing you to miss some time from family, work, school, or social activities.

Make an appointment **today** to discuss your HIT-6 results and your headaches with your doctor.

▼ **If You Scored 50 – 55**

Your headaches seem to be having some impact on your life. Your headaches should not make you miss time from family, work, school, or social activities.

Make sure you discuss your HIT-6 results and your headaches at your next appointment with your doctor.

▼ **If You Scored 49 or Less**

Your headaches seem to be having little to no impact on your life at this time. We encourage you to take HIT-6 monthly to continue to track how your headaches affect your life.

▼ **If Your Score on HIT-6 is 50 or Higher**

You should share the results with your doctor. Headaches that are disrupting your life could be migraine.

Take HIT-6 with you when you visit your doctor because research shows that when doctors understand exactly how badly headaches affect the lives of their patients, they are much more likely to provide a successful treatment program, which may include medication.

HIT is also available on the Internet at www.headachetest.com.

The Internet version allows you to print out a personal report of your results as well as a special detailed version for your doctor.

Don't forget to take HIT-6 again or try the Internet version to continue to monitor your progress.

▼ **About HIT**

The Headache Impact Test (HIT) is a tool used to measure the impact headaches have on your ability to function on the job, at school, at home and in social situations. Your score shows that the effect that headaches have on normal daily life and your ability to function. HIT was developed by an international team of headache experts from neurology and primary care medicine in collaboration with the psychometricians who developed the SF-36® health assessment tool.

HIT is not intended to offer medical advice regarding medical diagnosis or treatment. You should talk to your healthcare provider for advice specific to your situation.

SF-36® is a registered trademark of Medical Outcomes Trust and John E. Ware, Jr.

Useful websites

Websites for professionals
The British Association for the Study of Headache—www.bash.org.uk
This provides key guidelines for the management of headache which are UK specific and updated periodically.
American Headache Society—www.ahsnet.org
Offers a wide range of educational materials for professionals and patients. Also provides evidence-based reviews of the headache literature.
International Headache Society—www.i-h-s.org
Supports professionals working in the headache field and produces the International Classification of Headache Disorders which is available on the website.
Migraine in Primary Care Advisors— www.mipca.org.uk
Provides guidelines for the management of migraine in primary care.

Websites for patients
Migraine Action Association—www.migraine.org.uk
Migraine Trust –www.migrainetrust.org
The Organisation for the Understanding of Cluster Headache—www.ouchuk.org
World Headache Alliance—www.w-h-a.org
A cooperative of all lay headache organizations across the world providing information and support globally.

Patient consent form for occipital nerve injection

- Greater occipital nerve injection is a local procedure performed on the back of the head where this nerve crosses the scalp. The injection is a mixture of steroids and local anaesthetic.
- It is a therapeutic procedure performed as a short-term relief measure in patients with difficult to treat or very disabling headache.
- Side effects include tenderness at the injection point, transient dizziness and slight bleeding at the injection point.
- A rare side effect is (approximately 1%): lipatrophy (fat loss) at the injection site with loss of hair growth (~1p coin size). The hair may not grow back.

Statement of interpreter (where appropriate)

I have interpreted the information above to the patient/parent to the best of my ability and in a way in which I believe s/he/they can understand.

Signed................................Date........................

Name (print)........................

Statement of the patient/person with parental responsibility for the patient.

I agree to the procedure described above.

Signature..............................Date........................

Confirmation of consent

I have confirmed that the patient/parent has no further questions and wishes the procedure to go ahead.

Signature..............................Date........................

Name (print)........................Job Title........................

Some important drug interactions

These notes are for guidance only and are not exhaustive. Prescribers should refer to the manufacturer's data sheet. The prescriber should discuss the benefits and risks of each drug with the individual patient.

Drug	Interaction with	Notes
TRIPTANS	MAO inhibitors	Triptans metabolized via MAO. Potential for raised plasma concentrations of triptans
	Ergotamine, Ergot derivatives including methylsergide	Additive effect. Contraindicated.
	SSRIs	Theoretical possibility of serotonin syndrome (see page **)
Rizatriptan	Propranolol	Increases concentration of rizatriptan—use lower dose
Eletriptan	St John's Wort	Undesirable effects may be more common
Almotriptan	Itraconazole Ketoconazole	Raised plasma concentration, risk of toxicity
Eletriptan	Ketoconazole	Raised plasma concentration, risk of toxicity
Zolmitriptan	Protease inhibitors, e.g. indinavir, nelfinavir, ritonavir	Risk of toxicity, plasma concentration increased
	CYP 3A4 inhibitors, e.g. ketoconazole, itraconazole, erythromycin, clarithromycin	
	Cimetidine	Metabolism inhibited by cimetidine, with increased plasma levels
β-BLOCKERS	Other hypotensive agents	Hypotensive effect increased.
	Interaction with anti arrhythmics	Increased myocardial depression particularly verapamil
	Interaction with ergot alkaloids	Increased peripheral vasoconstriction
Propranolol	Rizatriptan	Increases plasma concentration of rizatriptan—reduce dose

Continued

Drug	Interaction with	Notes
Labetalol Metopranolol Propranolol	Cimetidine	Increased plasma concentration
TCAs	Alcohol	Increases sedative effect
	Tramadol and other opiates	Increases sedative effect
	Antiarrhythmic drugs	Increased risk of arrhythmia
	Antiepileptics	Antagonize anticonvulsant effect
	Lithium	Risk of toxicity
SODIUM VALPROATE	Aspirin	Effect of sodium valproate enhanced
	Erythromycin	Effect of sodium valproate enhanced
	Olanzapine	Risk of neutropenia
	Diazepam and lorazepam	Sodium valproate increases plasma concentration
	Cimetidine	Increased plasma concentration of sodium valproate
TOPIRAMATE	Carbamazepine	Concentration of topiramate reduced
	Oestrogens and progestogens	Topiramate accelerates metabolism of oestrogens and progestogens with reduced contraceptive effect
	Digoxin	Reduces digoxin plasma levels
	Thiazide diuretics	Potential increase in plasma concentration of topiramate
	Metformin	Potential for interaction. Monitor glucose
VERAPAMIL	Digoxin	Digoxin level increased
	β-Blockers and other arrhythmic agents	AV block bradycardia hypotension heart failure. Avoid
	Carbamazepine, Ciclosporin, Theophyline	Plasma levels of theses drugs increased
	Phenytoin, Phenobarbital	Verapamil levels reduced
	Lithium	Levels of lithium may be reduced, with an increased sensitivity to lithium causing neurotoxicity
	Cimetidine	Increase in verapamil level

Drug	Interaction with	Notes
DOMPERIDONE	Opiate analgesics	Antagonizes gastrointestinal activity
	CYP3 A4 inhibitors	May increase plasma levels of domperidone but unlikely to be relevant for single doses

Dermatomes and cranial nerves

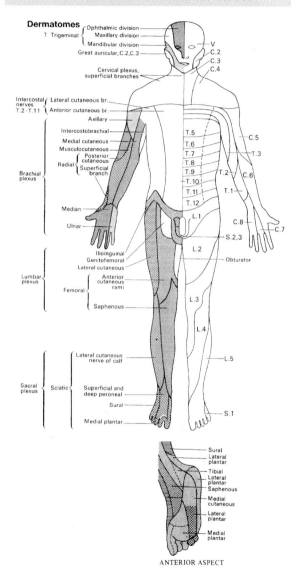

Dermatomes

T Trigeminal — Ophthalmic division
Maxillary division
Mandibular division
Great auricular, C.2, C.3

V
C.2
C.3
C.4

Cervical plexus, superficial branches

Intercostal nerves T.2–T.11 — Lateral cutaneous br.
Anterior cutaneous br.
Axillary
Intercostobrachial
Medial cutaneous
Musculocutaneous
Posterior cutaneous
Radial — Superficial branch
Median
Ulnar

Brachial plexus

T.5
T.6
T.7
T.8
T.9
T.10
T.11
T.12

C.5
T.3
T.2
C.6
T.1
C.8
C.7

L.1

Lumbar plexus — Ilioinguinal
Genitofemoral
Lateral cutaneous
Anterior cutaneous rami
Femoral — Saphenous

S.2,3
L.2
Obturator
L.3
L.4
L.5

Sacral plexus — Sciatic — Lateral cutaneous nerve of calf
Superficial and deep peroneal
Sural
Medial plantar

S.1

Sural
Lateral plantar
Tibial
Lateral plantar
Saphenous
Medial cutaneous
Lateral plantar
Medial plantar

ANTERIOR ASPECT

Reproduced from Longmore et al.(2004). *Oxford Handbook of Clinical Medicine*, 6th edition. Oxford University Press.

Dermatomes

Ophthalmic division
Maxillary division } Trigeminal
Mandibular division

Mastoid branch, C.2, C.3 } Superficial
Great auricular branch, C.2, C.3 } cervical plexus

Occipital, C.2
Occipital, C.3 } Dorsal
Occipital, C.4 } branches
Occipital, C.5-C.8

Supraclavicular, C.3, C.4

Dorsal rami of thoracic nerves

Cutaneous branch of axillary

Lateral cutaneous branches
of intercostal nerves

Medial and lateral cutaneous br. of radial

Medial cutaneous

Intercostobrachial

Musculocutaneous

Anterior branch of radial

Median

Dorsal cutaneous branch of ulnar

Gluteal branch of 12th intercostal

Lateral cutaneous br. of iliohypogastric

Lateral branches of dorsal
rami of lumbar and sacral

Medial branches of dorsal rami, L.1–S.6

Perforating branch of } Pudendal plexus
Posterior cutaneous }

Lateral cutaneous
Obturator
Medial cutaneous } Femoral } Lumbar plexus
Saphenous }

Posterior cutaneous

Superficial peroneal } Common
Sural } peroneal } Sacral plexus

Tibial

Lateral plantar

POSTERIOR ASPECT

Reproduced from Longmore et al.(2004). *Oxford Handbook of Clinical Medicine*, 6th edition. Oxford University Press.

Further reading

Carolei A, et al. (1996). History of migraine and risk of cerebral ischaemia in young adults. *Lancet.* **347**: 1503–6.

Chang C, et al. (1999). Migraine and stroke in young women: case-control study. *BMJ.* **318**: 13–8.

Goadsby, PJ, Dodick, D and Silberstein, SD (2005). *Chronic Daily Headache for Clinicians.* Hamilton, Canada: BC Decker Inc.

Headache Classification Committee of The International Headache Society (2004). The International Classification of Headache Disorders (second edition). *Cephalalgia*, **24**, 1–160.

Lance, JW and Goadsby, PJ (2005). *Mechanism and Management of Headache.* New York: Elsevier.

Lipton, RB and Bigal, M (2006). *Migraine and Other Headache Disorders.* New York: Marcel Dekker, Taylor & Francis Books, Inc.

Olesen, J, Tfelt-Hansen, P, Ramadan, N, Goadsby, PJ and Welch, KMA (2005). *The Headaches.* Philadelphia: Lippincott, Williams & Wilkins.

Silberstein, SD, Lipton, RB, Goadsby, PJ and Smith, RT (1999). *Headache in Primary Care.* Oxford: Isis Medical Media.

Silberstein, SD, Lipton, RB and Goadsby, PJ (2002). *Headache in Clinical Practice.* London: Martin Dunitz.

Silberstein, SD, Lipton, RB and Dodick, D (2008). *Wolff's Headache and Other Head Pain.* New York: Oxford University Press.

Tzourio C, et al. (1995). Case-control study of migraine and risk of ischaemic stroke in young women. *BMJ.* **310**: 830–3.

Index